STAGE-BY-STAGE
BABY FOOD COOKBOOK

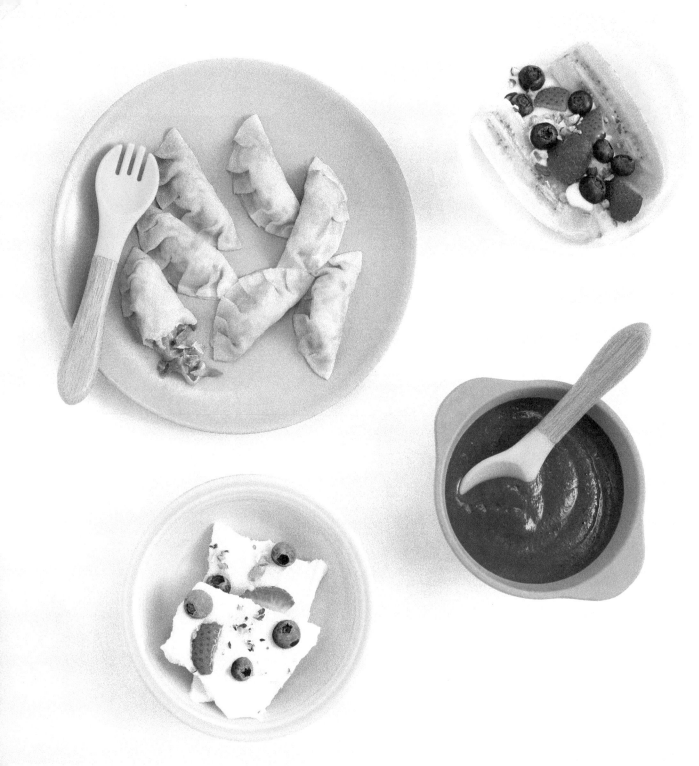

Stage-by-Stage

BABY FOOD COOKBOOK

100+ PURÉES AND
BABY-LED FEEDING RECIPES
FOR A HEALTHY START

BY YAFFI LVOVA, RDN
PHOTOGRAPHY BY LAURA FLIPPEN

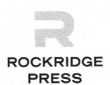

ROCKRIDGE
PRESS

For general information on our other products and services or to obtain technical support, please contact our Customer Care Department within the United States at (866) 744-2665, or outside the United States at (510) 253-0500.

Interior & Cover Designer: Linda Snorina
Art Producer: Sue Bischofberger
Editor: Laura Apperson
Production Editor: Nora Milman
Photography © 2019 Laura Flippen.
Author photo courtesy of Crystal Clear Photography.

Cover (from left to right): Cherry, Apple, and Sweet Corn Yogurt Pops; Carrot, Sweet Potato, and Brown Rice Purée; Sweets and Beets; Flatbread Pizza

ISBN: Print 978-1-64152-971-6 | eBook 978-1-64152-972-3

R0

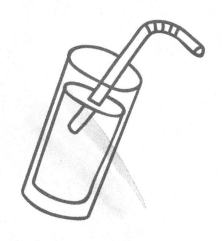

THIS IS FOR THE NEW PARENT.
I RAISE MY GLASS (OF MILK) TO YOU.
YOU ARE RAISING THE NEXT
GENERATION OF FOOD LOVERS.

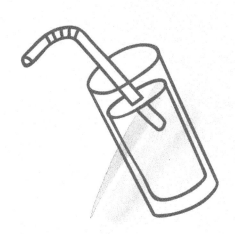

CONTENTS

3

4

5

12 TO 18 MONTHS

EARLY TODDLER GUIDE AND RECIPES 113

6

FAMILY FOOD GUIDE AND RECIPES 151

INTRODUCTION

Welcome to *Stage-by-Stage Baby Food Cookbook*! If you're reading this, you're either considering introducing food to your baby and looking for solid, reliable advice, or you've started introducing food and realized that there is a lot of confusing information out there. Perhaps you're way more ahead of the game than I ever was—you're expecting a baby and planning for all the beautiful milestones to come.

I'm Yaffi Lvova, a registered dietitian nutritionist and the owner of Baby Bloom Nutrition® and Toddler Test Kitchen™. I never thought I would be here, writing to you about how to feed your baby. I never thought there was all that much to it—until I had my twins. Picture this: two six-month-old babies attached to opposite sides of a long table in table-gripping baby seats and me running with a spoon between them. As if I had had enough sleep for that kind of workout. My whole nutrition practice is about helping you, the new parent, glide more gracefully into parenthood than I did.

In this book, I use a combination of personal and clinical experience, along with formal nutrition education and current research, to provide moderate, practical, and easy-to-follow advice that's backed up by recommendations from the American Academy of Pediatrics and the Academy of Nutrition and Dietetics. As your child begins to experience the flavor and texture of their first foods, you can interact on a new level, introducing your baby to your family traditions and culture. I'm here to guide you to a place where you can enjoy this exciting time with your family. There are very few hard rules to follow:

* Introduce solid food around six months old.

* Avoid choking hazards.

* Reduce salt before 12 months old.

* No milk to drink and no honey before 12 months old.

* Never leave your baby alone with food.

That's about it.

Two very common methods of food introduction are purées and baby-led feeding (also called baby-led weaning). This book takes a middle-of-the-road approach, recognizing that each option has its own benefits, develops oral muscles and fine motor skills in unique ways, and exposes your baby to different flavors and textures. I encourage you to find a sweet spot where your baby will progress in food enjoyment while you remain comfortable and enjoy the process along with your little one. Whether you choose baby-led feeding, purées, or a combination of the two, I'll guide you through the stages of infant development while providing easy and delicious recipes for the whole family.

Beginning in chapter 5, you'll start to see references to cooking with your children. The best thing you can do for your kids' health is to create happy memories around food and movement. Cook together, talk to them about groceries while shopping, and join them in unplanned avocado facials. By providing a variety of food experiences beyond just eating, you will give your baby will gain important exposure to different flavors, textures, and smells. The more familiar your baby is with a wide array of food sensory experiences, the more open they will be to trying new foods as they grow.

The single ingredient that should be present in every meal is joy.

Now let's get started!

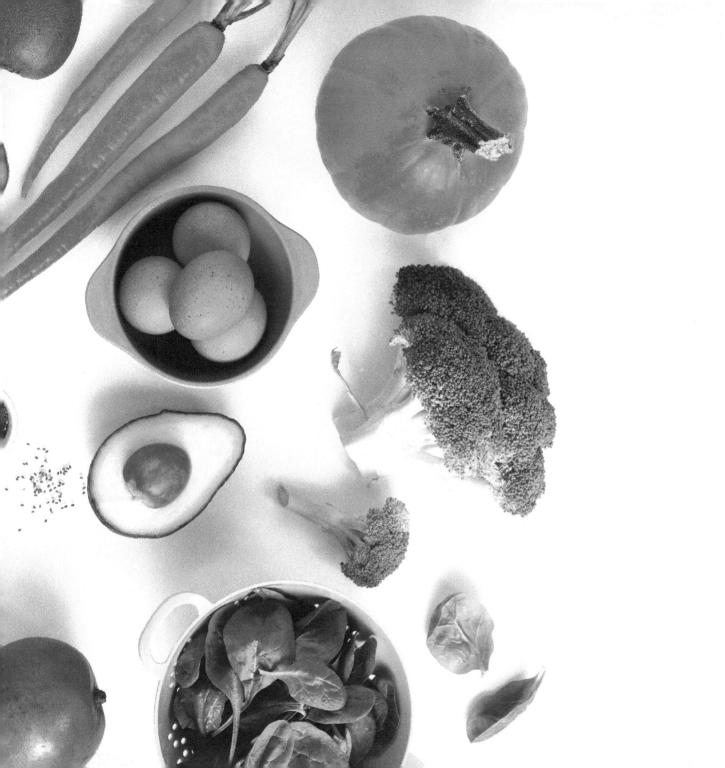

A HEALTHY START TO SOLIDS

You've noticed your baby eyeing your plate and maybe even trying to grab a bite of your food. Being able to share your love of food with your child is so exciting. But are you ready? Is your baby ready? How do you know what to provide first? Or how to prepare it? Do you need to start with purées? What about baby cereal? Let's jump in.

AN EXCITING MILESTONE

When you and your baby are both ready, this introduction to food will be an enjoyable and playful time.

IS YOUR BABY READY FOR SOLIDS?

At just around six months, but usually not earlier, your baby will start to show an interest in food. They will eye your plate, carefully observe you as you eat, and possibly reach for something delicious.

You'll know that your baby is ready when they display specific signs that indicate their digestive tract is ready to take in and absorb food safely. Here are some things your baby will do to show they're ready for solids:

- Show interest in food

- Physically move food from the front of the mouth to the back without pushing it out

- Attempt chewing or gumming food

- Work toward their pincer grasp (a skill that won't be perfected until around nine months)

- Sit up without assistance

ARE YOU READY?

To enjoy this magical time with your baby, it's important to be in touch with your own feelings about food. Often, introducing food can bring up a parent's previous (or current) food relationship struggles. Your goal is to teach your baby all about food enjoyment. This process will require a change in routine and schedules, and no matter which food introduction method you choose, there will be some mess involved. It's all part of the fun, but you can truly be present in the moment by preparing for this inevitability. If you feel that your family may benefit from some personalized guidance, there are pediatric dietitians who can help you and your baby move forward through this fun and exciting time.

There are very few hard-and-fast rules when it comes to food introduction, and there are many safe paths to take, whether you choose purées, baby-led feeding, or a combination of the two. When safety comes first and joy follows as a close second, your baby will learn to enjoy a variety of foods, which will benefit them for years to come.

WHY STAGE BY STAGE?

The difference between a six-month-old and a nine-month-old is startling. With each month, your baby grows, develops new skills, and enjoys new experiences.

STAGE-BY-STAGE PURÉES

You may be familiar with baby food stages, but if you wait for the readiness signs that appear around the six-month mark, you don't need to divide puréed foods into stages. Your six-month-old baby can safely enjoy thin, smooth purées just as well as thicker foods with more texture. This book is structured into stages in your child's development, such as your child's transition from palmar to pincer grasp, which brings the ability to manage different sizes and types of foods. It is of utmost importance that you as the parent feel safe and confident in food introduction, so if you prefer to move from thin purées into thicker textures rather than try it all at once, this book is a resource for those transitions as well.

Purées became popular in post–World War II America. In "Booming Baby Food: Infant Food and Feeding in Post–World War II America," Amy Bentley states that the standard advice during that time was to start babies on puréed foods at around six weeks of age. A child that age can't possibly pick up, gum, or swallow anything other than thin purées placed at the very back of the tongue. As a result, early feeding has been associated with an increased risk for choking (as the very young baby can't move their neck to manage the spit-up of partially digested foods) as well as an increased risk for food allergies, obesity, inadequate growth and development, and other health concerns. By watching for the readiness signs around six months, you can be sure that your child has reached a developmental stage where it is safe to introduce foods. Until then, continue feeding your baby breast milk or formula, and refer back to this book, where you'll be guided through each stage.

BABY-LED FEEDING

Baby-led feeding, also called baby-led weaning, is a method of food introduction that allows you to skip purées altogether and opt for an inclusive eating style. Despite its name, this method has nothing to do with breastfeeding cessation. This family-integrated dining experience provides the baby with the same food that the rest of the family is eating, in largely the same form. The baby self-feeds, enjoying the opportunity to develop fine motor skills and improve oral muscular movements while benefiting from being exposed to textures and flavors alongside the rest of the family.

Another benefit of baby-led feeding is more consistent food exposure. Although purées contain nutrients and flavor, the physical appearance of the food is so changed that the food won't be recognized when it's eventually served whole. When foods are given in their whole form, they are easily recognized, which positively impacts future acceptance.

If you choose baby-led feeding, it's beneficial to introduce foods by stages that align with your child's advances in fine motor skills, beginning with the palmar grasp and transitioning to the pincer grasp that's needed for smaller pieces. Additionally, foods given to your baby should contain very little salt, since your baby's kidneys are not ready to process much salt before 12 months, and the temperature of the food should be appropriate for little hands and mouths.

If you wait until the readiness signs that appear around the six-month mark, your main concern will be what you can confidently provide. Once feeding is developmentally appropriate, a baby can handle a variety of textures, flavors, and ingredients.

THIS BOOK'S FEEDING PHILOSOPHY

The feeding philosophy encouraged in this book is a combination of purées and baby-led feeding. A family may choose baby-led feeding or purées based on a number of valid factors, including schedule, family dynamic, culture, and personal comfort. Puréed meals are more efficient and (sometimes) less messy, and they work different muscles than whole foods. Baby-led feeding, on the other hand, doesn't require you to prepare or purchase additional food beyond what you are already buying and preparing for your family. Baby-led feeding also encourages whole-food recognition, which can help your family avoid certain selective (picky) eating concerns in the future.

Food introduction can be seen as a spectrum with purées on one side and baby-led feeding on the other; it's fine to be anywhere on that spectrum. Each family can find the dynamic that works best for them.

THE IMPORTANCE OF SCHEDULES AND ROUTINES

Children thrive within healthy boundaries. A predictable schedule and consistent routine will help a young child cope with transitions throughout the day. A regular schedule can also help an overwhelmed parent feel more confident.

When you first introduce food, treat it as a time for exploration and enjoyment. Just like a parent might expect a child to bang on a piano but not play anything recognizable, you should keep your expectations at a minimum during this new stage.

As your baby gets older, a predictable meal routine can help ensure their confidence at the table. This confidence can lead to an adventurous outlook on food as well as a feeling of self-assuredness in other areas of the child's life.

As you create your routine, serve meals and snacks two to three hours apart beginning at six months and into the early childhood years. This schedule allows your child's appetite to grow without letting them experience intense hunger. To assist you as you develop a routine, sample schedules will appear at the beginning of each of the following chapters.

FEEDING YOUR BABY THE FIRST YEAR

As you progress through this book, stage-specific information will guide you safely and confidently through this journey with your child.

MAINTAIN BREAST MILK OR FORMULA

Have you heard the saying "Food before one is just for fun"? Although primary nutrition before the 12-month mark comes from breast milk or formula, food plays a large role in exposing your baby to textures and flavors, developing their oral muscles, and letting them observe your social behavior modeling.

Breast milk or formula is complete and perfect until six months and remains a wonderful source of nutrition to two years and beyond. After six months, your baby also needs iron, zinc, and vitamin D. Babies are commonly given fruits and vegetables to supply these nutrients. Though fruits and vegetables provide many micronutrients, they lack fat and protein. Nutrition provided by breast milk or formula meets a baby's needs much more effectively than solid food does at this age. A baby cannot grow on vegetables alone!

As you begin introducing food to your baby, feed your baby breast milk or formula immediately prior to a solid meal to ensure that they are not actively hungry. Feeding at this stage is an activity, and hunger can be an overwhelming sensation that gets in the way. As your baby approaches eight to nine months, you can begin to space out liquid nutrition and solid nutrition to allow the baby to develop an appetite, but don't give them solid foods (including purées) less than 45 minutes before the breast or bottle or you'll risk interfering with their appetite for the next liquid meal.

INTRODUCE SOLIDS AT SIX MONTHS

The current recommendations from the American Academy of Pediatrics state that solid food—all foods other than breast milk or formula—should be introduced around six months old and that a variety of foods and textures should be included. This applies to both breast milk–fed and formula-fed babies. As your baby approaches that half-birthday, you'll notice their increased interest in food, as discussed earlier. As their tiny digestive tract matures, these outward signals show that the baby is ready for solids.

Introducing food too early has been associated with increased allergies, diabetes, inappropriate growth patterns, and aspiration (food or spit-up getting sucked into the airway). Introducing food too late brings the risk of slow growth, iron deficiency, delayed development of oral motor muscles, and an aversion to solid foods.

OFFER APPROPRIATE FOODS AND FLAVORS

If you've chosen baby-led feeding, you can give your baby nearly any food that the family enjoys. Remember, foods should be low in salt, easy to grab and tailored to the baby's grasping skills, and served cold or at room temperature to slightly warm. There is no reason to fear traditionally "adult" foods, such as sushi or dishes with complex flavors. Babies around the world enjoy vastly different flavors, so be encouraged to try something you may not have considered.

Avoid choking hazards until four years of age, including these foods:

* Whole nuts and hard seeds

* Hot dogs

* Whole grapes, grape tomatoes, cherry tomatoes

* Hard, gooey, and stick candy, including taffy, gum, and marshmallows

* Certain raw vegetables and fruits, including carrots and apples

* Chunks of nut or seed butter

* Chunks of meat or cheese

* Raisins and dried cranberries

* Fish with bones

* Popcorn

If you've chosen to go with purées as a first food, the world is your oyster. You can buy premade baby food or you can try the healthy and delicious recipes in this book. Purées can be simple or complex. They can be smooth or chunky. They can also be introduced in different ways. As you make these daily decisions, this book will help you remain confident that you're doing the best for your baby.

Purée pouches are great when you're on the go or in a pinch, but your baby's exposure to food should not be limited to them. The oral muscle work involved when consuming a pouch of puréed food is exactly the same as the sucking action used when feeding from the breast or bottle. Your baby has had six months to master that skill, and it's time to learn something new.

A great way to help your baby self-feed while using purées is to use the loaded-spoon method. Load the spoon with puréed food and place the spoon in front of your baby. If they want to play with the spoon, have a second spoon on hand—one for holding and one for eating.

If you choose to spoon-feed your baby, there are a couple of points to keep in mind:

MIND YOUR PACE: Wait for your child to lean forward and open their mouth before providing a bite.

PAY ATTENTION TO YOUR BABY'S CUES: When your baby purses their lips, turns their head sideways, or starts throwing food, the meal is over. These actions indicate that they are no longer interested in eating at this time. You respecting this, regardless of the amount of food consumed or left over, will help your child understand that their nutrition intake is dictated by their internal cues. This understanding can help your child maintain a positive relationship with food and with their body through childhood and into adulthood.

WATCH FOR REACTIONS

The benefit of baby-led feeding is that your baby will feed themselves to meet their appetite. If you have chosen to go with purées or a combination of methods, watch for your baby's reactions to ensure a comfortable feeding adventure for all.

Just as infants signal that they're hungry by rooting and that they're full by turning away from the breast or the bottle, a six-month-old child will display similar signs. A child who would like another bite will lean toward the spoon with an open mouth. The child may clap, laugh, hum, or make other pleasant noises. A child who is finished with the meal, regardless of the exact amount consumed, will turn their head, smear food on their tray, or throw something. These are not signs of poor behavior or acting out but rather the child's way of communicating their appetite. The best way forward is to remove the child from the seat and move on with the next activity.

Whether you've chosen purées or baby-led feeding, you'll notice your baby gagging. Unlike an adult's, a baby's gag reflex is triggered at the front of their mouth and teaches them the appropriate bite size and how to move food around their mouth. Gagging is a normal part of learning to eat, just as falling is a normal part of learning to walk. Remain calm when this reaction occurs so that your baby does not associate fear with eating. But you should learn first aid for choking in the rare case that your baby does begin to choke.

INCREASE SOLIDS GRADUALLY

Food introduction should be a fun and exciting time for parent and child alike. If your baby is too tired or too hungry, if the atmosphere is too loud, if you're too close or too exuberant, the child may feel overwhelmed and overstimulated. Start slowly and increase solids gradually to avoid overstimulation.

A fun way to imagine how your baby feels is to role-play with a partner: Take a turn

RAISING AN ADVENTUROUS EATER

Children are naturally curious, which is why, from 6 months until about 12 to 18 months, there is a golden opportunity to introduce new foods. Your baby will seize any chance to learn something new, usually by putting something in their mouth. As your baby develops and begins to walk, you may notice a shift in their interest in new foods as they tend to stick with what they know—the foods you have already introduced and made familiar.

Sensory processing differences may also affect a child's adventurous attitude. Sensory differences can range from sensory sensitivity to sensory processing disorder, which would be diagnosed by a pediatrician. When a child is sensitive to sensory input, the texture of an orange might feel painful, the crunch of a cracker might be overwhelming, and the smell of cooking food might be too much to handle. This sensitivity can impact a child's attitude at the table, since everything is a bit scarier than the parent intended. If your child is sensitive to sensory input, practice compassion and allow them space to explore without pressure or expectations. If their perception of smell, taste, and sound seems to interfere with their ability to enjoy food, discuss it with your pediatrician.

Food allergies or intolerances and a history of acid reflux may also impact a child's perspective of unfamiliar foods. If your child is limiting their food intake and decreasing the number of acceptable foods without trying new ones, you may want to consult a feeding therapist.

Maximize your child's sense of adventure by offering varied foods, avoiding pressure to eat a specific amount or item, and sitting with your child to enjoy something delicious together.

being the baby and describe to your partner how it feels. Overstimulation can be avoided with careful timing and by keeping a calm, relaxed atmosphere during mealtimes.

Throughout childhood, your baby's portion size will match the size of their fist. Seconds, and sometimes thirds, are always available as your child learns to respect their hunger and fullness cues. Giving small portions with access to more as their appetite indicates helps avoid overstimulation while also preventing excessive food waste. For consistency in this book, a purée serving size is two ounces.

When your child is around eight months old, you'll want to start developing a consistent meal and snack schedule. Starting sooner than that can help you with meal planning and staying organized with the daily schedule. Referring to the stage-by-stage guides in this book will help you feel confident and on track.

A BALANCED DIET FOR YOUR BABY

It's said that "variety is the spice of life." Providing a range of foods for your baby, while minding which few foods you should avoid, will give your baby the nutrition they need and set them up for future food acceptance and enjoyment.

NUTRIENTS BABIES NEED

In the first year, your baby's primary nutrition comes from breast milk or formula. Breast milk has the perfect ratio of fats, carbohydrates, and protein to meet a growing baby's needs. It also contains immune-supporting compounds. Breast milk changes over time, and even day by day, to meet the baby's needs. Formula production methods have come a very long way in imitating breast milk. Modern formulas are developed by teams of professionals, in sterile environments, to ensure the healthiest and safest nutrition.

Solid food intake begins at six months and provides three crucial nutrients: iron, zinc, and vitamin D. If your family consumes meat, you may introduce it among the first foods. Try giving your baby shredded chicken that's been slow cooked or a strip of steak (long enough to fit through the baby's fist and poke out the top). Just gumming these foods provides enough iron and zinc to meet your baby's needs at this stage.

Iron-rich plant foods include spinach, legumes, and quinoa, and several recipes in this book contain these ingredients. By pairing these foods with a fruit or vegetable high in vitamin C, while avoiding dairy in the same meal, you can maximize your child's iron absorption. If you're concerned about iron absorption, avoid serving dairy in meals that have high iron levels, as the calcium in dairy slows the absorption of iron. This interaction is only a concern when calcium and iron are consumed together.

Vitamin D and zinc are in fortified dairy products, such as yogurt and cheese. The American Academy of Pediatrics recommends a daily vitamin D dose of 400 IU for babies up to 12 months for a few reasons. Our main source of vitamin D is sunlight, but because of lifestyle factors and concern about skin cancer, we cover up our skin and are not able to naturally create the vitamin D levels our bodies need. Breast milk does not contain vitamin D, and the amount in most baby formulas is insufficient. Talk to your pediatrician before starting your baby on any new supplements.

FOODS TO LIMIT OR AVOID

Until your child is 12 months old, be sure to avoid these foods:

MILK: Cow's milk displaces important nutrition from breast milk or formula.

HONEY: Honey carries a risk of botulism, an illness caused by a bacterium that older children and adults can easily fight. Honey should never be given before your child is 12 months old, even in a cooked food.

SALT: Limit added salt during the first year as your baby's kidneys mature. After your baby reaches 12 months, you may opt to continue a lower-sodium lifestyle by using other seasonings, or you may prepare family recipes as you normally would. Sodium is found naturally in many foods but is also added to packaged foods as a preservative. Choose "low-sodium" or "no-salt-added" broths, canned goods, and other packaged foods when possible. Cheese is also a high-sodium food and should be limited to one meal per day.

FRUIT JUICE: Prune and pear juice can help with constipation. Start with two ounces for your baby. Otherwise, all fruit juice should be avoided.

HOW MUCH WATER?

Hydration under six months comes exclusively from breast milk or formula, even in very hot weather. Breast milk and formula provide the proper amount of electrolytes that babies need, and they don't need water at or between meals. Formula or expressed breast milk can be given with meals in a sippy cup or an open cup.

When a baby under six months old drinks water, their electrolyte balance may be thrown off, sometimes with dire consequences. This imbalance is called water intoxication and results when water lost through diarrhea, vomiting, sweating, or even urination is replaced with fluid that does not contain electrolytes. Water intoxication most often occurs when formula is made using too much water, but it can also happen when a child is given water rather than breast milk or formula.

ALLERGIES, INTOLERANCES, AND SENSITIVITIES

Food reactions such as coughing, wheezing, or swollen lips and tongue should be addressed immediately. Some children become constipated or have diarrhea after solid foods are introduced. Bowel habit changes are common and should only last a few days. Some children will react to a food with eczema or a rash around the mouth or in the diaper area. Some children may show hives or welts. Reactions can indicate a food intolerance or allergy, and they can be mild or more serious. Discuss any reaction with your pediatrician.

Food allergies can be passed through families. However, what is passed from one generation to the next isn't a specific food allergy but rather an increased risk the child will react to any food. For example, if one of the parents is allergic to seafood, your baby may have an increased risk for a food allergy but not necessarily to seafood. Talking to a pediatric dietitian or your pediatrician can help you feel confident about introducing potential allergens.

Here are the eight most common allergens, which cause 90 percent of all allergic reactions:

- Cow's milk
- Soy
- Eggs
- Wheat
- Peanuts
- Tree nuts (Note: Coconut is not included in this allergen, as most people who

are allergic to tree nuts can safely eat coconut.)

- Shellfish

- Fish

Current research shows that these foods should be introduced as soon as food introduction begins to minimize the chance of a reaction later on.

If introducing allergenic foods causes anxiety, time these introductions to coincide with a well-check at the pediatrician's office. Smear your baby's gums with a tiny bit of peanut butter before getting out of the car for the well-check. If there's an allergic reaction, the child is already in a place where it can be handled effectively and quickly.

If there is no family history of food allergies, you can introduce foods by giving your baby what the rest of the family is eating. If there is a significant history in the immediate family, you may choose to take a more cautious route. Introduce low-allergenic foods two to three days apart. Introduce higher allergenic foods (the eight most common allergens) one week apart with nothing new introduced during that week. This spacing allows time to check for a reaction to an unfamiliar food.

Intolerances and sensitivities are not the same as allergies. Food allergies are immune system responses to food proteins, while intolerances and sensitivities are nonimmune reactions. These reactions can be immediate or delayed. Symptoms may include gas, constipation, diarrhea, nausea, and headaches. Well-known food intolerances include lactose and gluten. These reactions will not be picked up with a standard allergy test. If you suspect a food reaction, discuss it with your pediatric dietitian.

BABY FOOD BUILDING BLOCKS

Is it time to start feeding your baby? Have you glanced in your refrigerator and your cabinets and now you're overwhelmed? Don't overthink it! What your baby needs right now is a colorful and varied experience that's free from stress so they can just enjoy their time with you.

COLORFUL FRUITS AND VEGETABLES

The various bright colors in fruits and vegetables represent different nutrients, flavors, and textures. The red in an apple is different than the red in a pepper. The foods taste different, feel different, and can even sound different. Whether you've chosen purées, baby-led feeding, or a combination, there are a wealth of options for your baby's first foods.

A VARIETY OF PROTEINS

Your baby's protein needs are being met with breast milk or formula, so you don't need to stress about protein intake. Providing your baby with different foods helps make the foods familiar, which will diminish the later selective (picky) phase. Many children actively avoid meat, as it tastes dry to them. This book has recipes and tips to address your child's avoidance of meat, or you can choose other protein-rich options. Beans, nuts, and eggs are great sources of protein, with nuts also providing brain-boosting fats.

FIBER-RICH WHOLE GRAINS

Fiber-rich whole grains provide protein, B vitamins, and antioxidants, as well as iron, magnesium, zinc, and copper. Whole grains are perfectly digested and absorbed at this stage. Lightly toasted whole-grain bread with a small smear of peanut butter or Burst

Tomatoes and Pasta (page 171) are both great sources of whole grains.

HEALTHY FATS AND OILS

Many packaged purées lack healthy fats and oils. When preparing homemade purées or choosing food for baby-led feeding, select foods high in anti-inflammatory fat. Fat is important for brain growth and development, energy, and the absorption of vitamins A, D, E, and K. You can include fat in your baby's meals by cooking with extra-virgin olive oil and by serving avocado, fatty fish (salmon, mackerel, sardines, and herring), cheese, full-fat yogurt, whole eggs, and nuts and seeds (ground or as nut butter). By serving baby foods that contain fats, you'll also be exposing your little one to more flavors.

FLAVORFUL HERBS AND SPICES

In many cultures, food is seasoned with herbs and spices, even spicy flavors. While your baby may or may not tolerate some cayenne pepper in their food, using basil, rosemary, garlic, cumin, and other seasonings can provide an amazing, flavorful

Parenting is a busy time. Here are some tips and tricks to help streamline your cooking process.

DO SOME LIGHT MEAL PREPARATION. By creating a plan, and a shopping list to go with that plan, you have options and the ingredients to make them happen. Meal prepping can mean anything from chopping vegetables to creating whole meals ahead of time. Find your groove and stick with it. You can easily meal prep by doubling a recipe and freezing half for later.

STOCK UP ON STAPLES. Rice, pasta, and frozen veggies all store well and make for a quick meal when you're short on time.

RELEASE THE PRESSURE VALVE. Not every food needs to be cooked from scratch. By choosing high-quality convenience items, such as hummus, crackers, and applesauce, you can have a variety of foods quickly available without additional effort. The increased time spent with your child, along with the reduction in stress, is essential for bonding with your baby.

REPURPOSE LEFTOVERS. You've already cooked it, so serve it up again or make it look like something new. Leftover grilled chicken breast can become fajitas. Leftover quinoa reappears as Quinoa Pizza Bites (page 49). And leftover mashed potatoes are perfect for Leftover Mashed Potato Soup (page 111)!

experience for your baby. A baby may not be interested in roasted butternut squash but with a sprinkle of cinnamon, it's a whole new experience. Consider adding basil to pasta, cumin to lentils, or cardamom to sweet potatoes.

ONLY THE BEST FOR YOUR BABY

Of course, you want to provide the best for your baby. But what does that mean? Let's clear up the confusion.

HOMEMADE VERSUS STORE-BOUGHT

You'll see many different types of baby food in the supermarket. Containers, ingredients, and prices vary, and it can be overwhelming. The thought of making baby food at home can also stir up some anxiety. But much like any other aspect of parenting, the choice you make doesn't have to be a permanent one. If you try something and it doesn't work for you and your family, you can make a different choice the next day. And you can always mix it up, serving both homemade and store-bought food.

Store-bought baby food has a very smooth texture and includes multiple ingredients, which can take a lot of energy to achieve at home. But creating food at home from whole, fresh ingredients comes with a sense of accomplishment and adventure. And some variety in texture comes with its own benefits as your baby learns to use their tongue to eat effectively.

ORGANIC VERSUS CONVENTIONAL

When deciding between organic and conventional produce, there are many factors to consider. Certain foods, such as bananas and avocados, are not as affected by pesticides because they have thick skins. Other plants are more susceptible: generally, plants with thin skins, such as peppers, tomatoes, and fruits with pits. Although it's nice to buy organic, research has shown that when weighing the risk of pesticides against the benefit of eating fruits and vegetables daily, a nutrition plan rich in plants is best, whether the produce is conventional or organic.

WHOLE FOODS VERSUS PROCESSED

By using a combination of store-bought and homemade baby food, you can enjoy the convenience of premade food and the ingredient control and lower price of homemade food. When looking at premade baby food, you may notice that although no commercially available baby food contains added sugar (as in table sugar), some may contain concentrated juice, which, effectively, is sugar. The truth is that babies and young children have extremely sensitive taste buds. They can pick up on, and enjoy, subtle flavors that adults miss. Added sweetness isn't at all necessary, and you can limit it by making homemade food or checking the ingredients list on a premade product.

THE BOTTOM LINE FOR GOOD HEALTH

When introducing solid food to your baby, variety in texture, color, and flavor are key. So, whether you choose store-bought or homemade, purées or baby-led feeding, your baby will experience the greatest benefit from the combination of variety and a pleasant table atmosphere—fun time with you!

HELPFUL TOOLS AND EQUIPMENT

Let's get cooking! You only need the basics to start, but as you gain confidence and expand your recipe Rolodex (or Pinterest board), you can always add some fancier tools.

COOKING TOOLS

Having the right tools on hand will help you get food on the table effectively and with minimal stress. Here are some tools that are beneficial for the recipes in this book.

Kitchen Basics

- **POTATO MASHER:** This handy tool can mash potatoes, but it's also great for making egg salad, guacamole, and applesauce.

- **ROLLING PIN:** From mini to standard size, tapered to handled, rolling pins come in many forms. If you don't have one on hand, you can always use a wine bottle.

- **SLOTTED SPOON:** Use this convenient tool for stirring and straining pasta and veggies.

- **PASTRY BRUSH:** Use a pastry brush to add a wash or a glaze to a baked good or meat or to spread oil or butter. When your little one is around 12 months old, you can let them use the brush to help you "paint" the food.

- **WHISK:** If you're stirring, blending, aerating, or whipping, a whisk is your friend. Get a miniature one so little hands can copy yours!

- **STEAMER INSERTS:** Whether you make your own purées or go with baby-led feeding, you'll love having a steamer insert.

BASIC POTS: Keeping a variety of pots, including a stock pot, a medium-size pot, and a saucepan, on hand will mean you're prepared for any recipe. By using the appropriate pot, you can minimize the mess and maximize your time.

BASIC PANS: Keep a cast iron skillet, sauté pan, and wok in the kitchen. The cast iron skillet can be used on the stovetop and in the oven or on the grill, it cleans nicely, and it adds extra nutrition to your dish. A wok is extremely versatile and can function as a pot or a pan, as it cooks evenly and can handle a large quantity of food.

MINI ICE-POP MOLDS: Teething children love ice pops. So do toddlers, older kids, and adults!

MUFFIN TINS: Muffins are great for breakfast or snacks. Whether you choose full-size or miniature, it's best to have some tins on hand.

MEAT THERMOMETER: This tool helps ensure safety, but it also protects flavor and texture by making sure you don't overcook your food.

Appliances

ELECTRIC BEATERS OR ELECTRIC MIXER: Although mixing by hand can be a great workout, an electric model will get you a smoother product in less time. Electric mixers come in many models, so find what works best for you.

ELECTRIC PRESSURE COOKER, RICE COOKER, OR SLOW COOKER: Electric pressure cookers are easy to use and clean, and you can make anything from a supersize Japanese pancake to a full dinner in one machine. Rice cookers can also cook other grains, as well as steam vegetables. A slow cooker lets you put your meal together, set it to cook, and forget it. If you're choosing among these three, the electric pressure cooker can perform the tasks of a rice cooker and a slow cooker.

IMMERSION BLENDER: If you're making homemade purées, this option will be much less pricey than some of the dedicated baby food machines. Simply cook your ingredients, then blend them in the same pot. An immersion blender is also a wonderful tool for making blended soups, sauces, and dips.

At six months, your baby still relies on breast milk or formula for most of their nutrition. Keeping that in mind, you don't need to stress over what to pack when leaving the house. Including a couple of purée pouches; a teething snack, such as Bamba; a veggie-based mini muffin; or some appropriately cut fruits or veggies will be perfect. As your baby gets older and you have a set routine for meals and snacks at home, you'll want to pack more food so you can stick as close as possible to your routine. Take some of the pressure off yourself by packing a combination of homemade and convenience items. If you're trying something new, serve something familiar along with it, and bring familiar snacks to an unfamiliar location. By reinforcing a consistent schedule and offering familiar food choices, you'll set you and your baby up for a pleasant adventure.

- **TOASTER OVEN:** This appliance will cook your food at the specified temperature and time and then turn itself off. A toaster oven is ideal for time-sensitive recipes that require an oven.

- **GRIDDLE:** It's almost impossible to burn something on an electric griddle, making it a must-have for new parents.

- **WAFFLE MAKER:** A waffle maker allows you to create tasty and nutritious waffles that can be frozen and reheated when you need them.

STORAGE EQUIPMENT

There are many options for storing and transporting your meals and snacks. But nobody wants a whole pile of dishes to clean after each outing! Bento boxes, which come in a multitude of styles, are easy to store in the fridge and easy to take with you. They have compartments for different types of food and they're solid, so your hard work won't get crushed in the diaper bag or the car. Bento boxes range in price, but inexpensive options are widely available.

For home use, any bowl that comes with a lid is your friend. Saving leftover chicken nuggets or storing excess hummus is easy in these containers.

FEEDING ESSENTIALS

Let's keep this simple because parenting, in general, isn't simple. You only need a few key essentials for starting solid foods with your baby.

- A **SOFT-TIPPED SPOON** is essential for safely feeding purées to your baby. When choosing baby-led feeding, opt for a spoon designed for self-feeding. This spoon will have a wider grip and often a shorter handle.

- Choose well-made **COLORFUL PLATES AND CUPS**. It's best to guide your child away from preferring separated foods by serving food on a nonsegmented plate. This approach may be different for a child with certain levels of sensory processing challenges, but in that case, you should follow the direction of your feeding specialist.

- The right **HIGH CHAIR** places your baby to your seated height, allows them to sit up straight, and provides foot support and an overall comfortable position.

- A **SIPPY CUP** with a soft spout will help your baby transition from the breast or bottle to an open cup. Experiment with an **OPEN CUP** at home. You can start transitioning to this cup as early as six months at the table and even earlier if your little one will be playing with it in the bathtub.

- **SILICONE FREEZER TRAYS** are very convenient for freezing homemade baby food. They are easy to use and easy to clean.

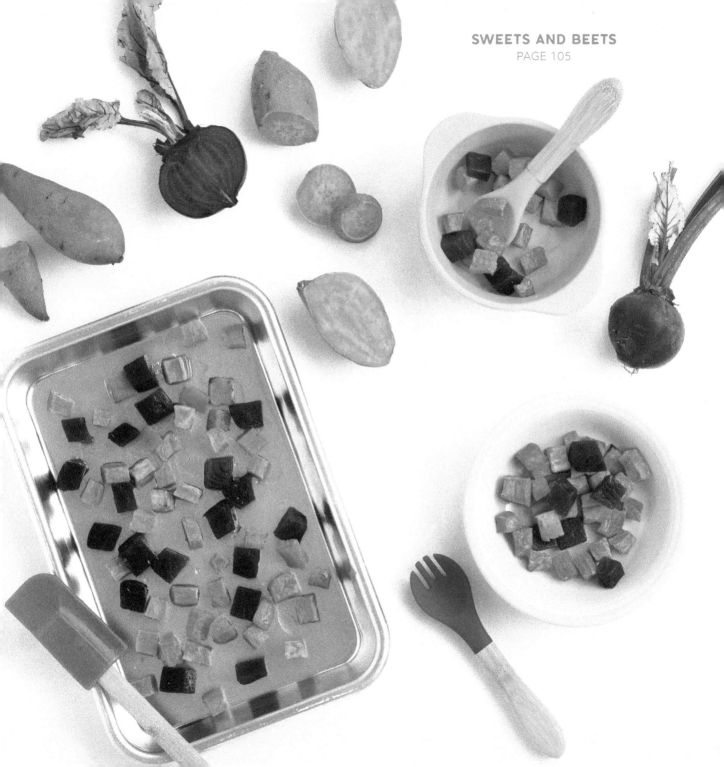

SWEETS AND BEETS
PAGE 105

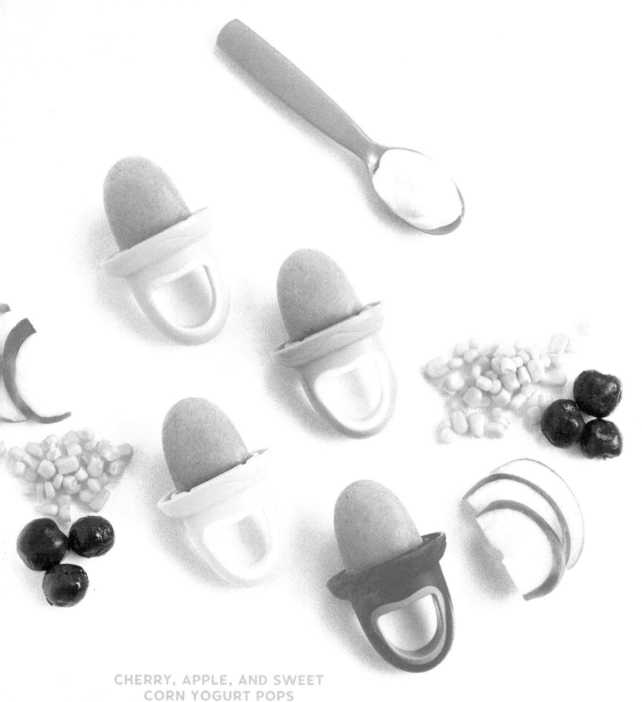

CHERRY, APPLE, AND SWEET
CORN YOGURT POPS
PAGE 38

AROUND 6 MONTHS
STAGE ONE GUIDE AND RECIPES

Your baby is about to turn six months old. Where has the time gone? Your baby is smiling, sitting up, and possibly even trying to crawl. They have been growing like a sprout, but their growth, both in weight and height, is going to slow a bit. As you begin to introduce solid foods, you'll notice that your baby's poop starts to change as well.

RECIPES 30

PURÉES

BABY-LED FEEDING

BABY AT THIS STAGE

"The only constant is change." This familiar saying is particularly apt during these early months of your baby's life. What can you begin to expect around six months?

DEVELOPMENTAL SKILLS

Around six months of age, your baby will likely have mastered the palmar grasp, using the whole fist to grab a toy or a piece of food. They will begin practicing the pincer grasp, but that is not expected to develop fully until closer to nine months. Appropriate use of utensils will be an ongoing and developing skill, but by introducing your baby to an age-appropriate fork and spoon early on, you can help them become familiar with that skill more quickly.

NUTRITIONAL NEEDS

Until now, breast milk or formula has been meeting most of your baby's nutritional needs. When your baby reaches six months of age, though, the iron stores in their liver, present from before birth, start to run low. Your baby needs to meet their iron and zinc requirements with solid food. They also need a vitamin D supplement, as discussed in chapter 1. Breast milk or formula remains the primary source of nutrition and should be continued until your baby is 12 months old, when milk or milk alternatives can safely replace it.

WHAT TO INTRODUCE

If you ask five people what to give your baby first, you'll get six different answers. What's the best advice? Don't overthink it!

FOODS AND FLAVORS

Any food you give your baby will be new and exciting. You don't need to spend valuable energy thinking too much about what to give them. Keep it simple so you can enjoy these foods alongside your child, sharing in the excitement together.

Here are some simple foods to try:

* Banana, either partially peeled or mashed

* Avocado, with a bit of peel still on for gripping or mashed with a fork

* Baked sweet potato, cut into wedges or mashed

* Soft steamed or roasted carrots

* Roasted zucchini spears

* Scrambled eggs

* Pear or peach wedges, peeled or mashed

* Steamed broccoli, in florets or mashed

If you've chosen baby-led feeding as a food introduction method, be sure to prepare the food in a way that allows your baby to effectively pick it up. For easier gripping, partially peel bananas and avocados so that the fruit is exposed at the top but some skin remains.

TOOLS AND UTENSILS

Specialized utensils aren't necessary but have some benefits that can make this process easier for you and less frustrating for your baby. You may want to try different options to see what works best for your family. When choosing utensils, these are the main features to look for:

- BPA-free

- Smooth edges

- Rounded fork ends

- Easy-grip handles

I like the NumNum GOOtensil because it has a wide grip and doesn't require balancing, so a baby can pick up a small amount of food at a time. The texture of the utensil is great for little gums that are sore from teething.

TYPICAL MEALS AND SCHEDULE

At six months, your baby is probably taking three or four naps per day. Your schedule might look something like the one below, although the times can be shifted as needed.

At this stage, your baby is awake for no more than two hours between naps and sticks to a routine of eat, play and sleep. See Resources (page 189) for more information on scheduling.

At mealtimes, the amount of food that makes it into your baby's belly isn't

6:00 A.M.	Wake and feed (breast milk or formula)
7:30 A.M.	Solid food breakfast
8:00 A.M.	Nap (45 to 60 minutes)
9:30 A.M.	Wake and feed (breast milk or formula)
10:00 A.M.	Snack option #1
11:00 A.M.	Nap (1½ to 2 hours or more)
1:00 P.M.	Wake and feed (breast milk or formula)
1:30 P.M.	Snack option #2
3:00 P.M.	Nap (20 to 60 minutes)
4:00 P.M.	Wake and feed (breast milk or formula)
4:30 P.M.	Solid food dinner
5:30 P.M.	Begin bedtime routine
6:30 P.M.	Breast milk or formula, then to bed

important, but providing too much food can be overwhelming, decreasing their interest. The portion size for any given food should be the size of the baby's fist. As your baby grows, their portion size will remain the size of their fist.

Feel free to give multiple portions, as your baby requests. As you respect your baby's appetite, they will learn that food is readily available. They can follow their instincts for how much to eat rather than be concerned there won't be enough food, which would cause them to overeat.

BABY'S FIRST FOOD!

Here are some guidelines for your baby's first food:

- Serve food cold to lukewarm.

- Offer food that is low in salt.

- Cut the food into sizes that are appropriate for gripping.

Additionally, choking hazards must be avoided, as mentioned in chapter 1.

Your baby experienced different flavors in the womb, as the foods you enjoyed actually flavored the amniotic fluid! Just as we can enjoy pizza and salad, your baby can enjoy both savory vegetables and sweet fruits, and the order in which foods are introduced has little to no impact on flavor preference.

You may mark this special occasion by getting your baby a new table, a nice placemat, age-appropriate utensils, and flowers to decorate the table. However, avoid overwhelming the child with too much fanfare, which may cause sensory overload and an uncomfortable experience for your child. Make sure the baby is fed by the breast or bottle prior to giving them solid or puréed food. As you get used to this routine, continue to refer to the sample feeding schedule for guidance.

COMMON CHALLENGES

ALLERGIES: If there is a significant history of family allergies, introduce new foods once every three days. For highly allergenic foods, wait a week between new food introductions. This spacing allows time to evaluate whether your baby has had a reaction and which food was the culprit.

GAGGING: This is a common worry, particularly for parents exploring baby-led feeding. As discussed in chapter 1, unlike an adult, who gags immediately before choking, a baby's gag merely indicates a large bite, causing the child to spit out the food and try again. Parents can temper their reaction by expecting gagging. Allow your child to work through this process on their own.

REASONABLE EXPECTATIONS: Between 6 and 12 months, food is important for oral muscular development, flavor and texture exposure, and social modeling. It is not important for nutrition, which is why you give your baby breast milk or formula prior to solid food meals until the one-year mark. A child may eat a lot at one meal and not much at the next. By viewing meals and snacks as an activity, much like a music class or playing with blocks, parents can keep their expectations appropriate and not worry about how much solid food their baby eats.

CONSTIPATION: A healthy baby will have at least one well-formed bowel movement per day, but at the start of solid food introduction, there may be a few days of adjustment. What you're putting in is changing, so what comes out will also be different. Monitor your baby for straining and crying during bowel movements, lack of appetite, refusal to eat, a hard belly, hard pellets in the diaper, or streaks of blood in the stool. There are some ways to help your baby through this time:

* **PATTERNS:** If constipation occurs when your baby eats a certain food, it may indicate a food sensitivity.

* **IRON:** Too much iron can cause constipation. Try switching out an iron-fortified food for a nonfortified version.

* **APPLES, PEARS, AND PRUNES:** Try out the Cinnamon Apples and Pumpkin (page 35) or Pear, Kiwifruit, and Spinach Purée (page 37).

* **TUMMY TIME:** Any activity on the stomach will help move things along.

* **TUMMY MASSAGE:** There are YouTube videos on infant massage for constipation.

* **BABYWEARING:** Strapping on your little one puts them in a position that mobilizes the tummy. The increased skin-on-skin contact also helps.

* **CHIROPRACTIC CARE:** Find a chiropractor who specializes in infant/baby care. Dr. Jolene Kuty of Kuty Chiropractic once told me: "In our chiropractic office, we sometimes tease that there should be a yellow triangle on the door that says, 'Beware, we may cause explosive poo-poo.'"

* **PROBIOTICS:** Look for a refrigerated powder containing at least four species or strains of bacteria, including lactobacillus and bifidobacterium. Following the package's instructions, mix the powder into a small amount of expressed breast milk, formula, or water, and use a syringe to give the mixture orally to your child. You can also mix it into a small amount of cottage cheese, yogurt, or smoothie.

My favorite probiotic for this age is Klaire Labs Ther-Biotic for Infants.

* **JUICE:** Try two ounces of 100 percent prune or pear juice. Although I don't recommend juice as part of a baby's nutrition, juices have proven to be successful for relieving constipation.

BROWN RICE

GLUTEN-FREE **NUT-FREE** VEGAN

YIELDS 9 SERVINGS

2 cups water
or low-sodium
vegetable broth

1 cup dried brown
rice, rinsed thoroughly

Brown rice is a whole-grain rice and a nutrition powerhouse that contains fiber, B vitamins, manganese, iron, and magnesium. It is a great first food for your baby and makes a great base for sweet or savory meals. Mix in purées for a full meal experience. Keep this recipe bookmarked—it will be used in a few different recipes!

1. Bring the water to a boil. Add the rinsed rice and return to a boil.

2. Reduce heat to low and cook for 50 minutes. Remove from heat and let stand for 10 minutes. Fluff with a fork to separate the rice grains.

STORAGE TIPS FOR ALL PURÉES:

TO REFRIGERATE: Store in a sealed container in the refrigerator for up to 5 days.

TO FREEZE: Portion into ice cube trays or a silicone baby food freezer tray. Freeze, then pop the cubes out and store in an airtight container for up to 3 months, removing each portion as needed. Defrost in one of three different ways:

- Let the purée thaw overnight in the fridge.
- Place sealed frozen bags of purées in a warm water bath until thawed.
- Place frozen baby food in a microwave-safe dish and use the defrost function on your microwave to thaw. Stir frequently and be sure that the food is the appropriate temperature prior to serving.

TO SERVE: Serve thawed baby food within 48 hours of defrosting. Discard any food that remains beyond that time.

OATMEAL WITH MIX-INS

GLUTEN-FREE   NUT-FREE   VEGAN

YIELDS 2 SERVINGS

1 cup old-fashioned oats

½ cup water

Mix-ins of your choice

It's common to start babies off with rice cereal, but oatmeal has all the same benefits with increased nutrition. Oatmeal is a great base for mix-ins and adds texture and body to any simple purée. It can be served smooth or a bit chunky for added texture exposure. You can certainly buy baby oatmeal, but grinding your own oats may be more economical. The leftover ground oats from this recipe can be kept in a sealed container in the refrigerator for up to a month.

1. Put the oats in a blender or food processor and pulse until ground. Measure out 2 tablespoons and store the remainder for later.

2. Bring the water to a boil. Add the 2 tablespoons of ground oatmeal to the boiling water.

3. Stir until thick, about 4 minutes.

4. Stir in mix-ins of your choice:
   a. Breast milk or formula to cool or thin
   b. ½ teaspoon of cinnamon
   c. ½ teaspoon of pumpkin pie spice
   d. 1 tablespoon of Cinnamon Apples and Pumpkin (page 35)
   e. 1 tablespoon of Pear, Kiwifruit, and Spinach Purée (page 37)

CARROT, CORN, AND PUMPKIN PURÉE

GLUTEN-FREE **NUT-FREE** VEGAN

YIELDS 6 SERVINGS

½ cup sweet
corn, steamed

4 ounces full-fat
canned coconut milk

8 ounces
carrots, steamed

½ cup
canned pumpkin

This recipe combines three naturally sweet foods to create a delicious introduction to some of our favorite seasonal vegetables. Using canned pumpkin reduces preparation time and makes the recipe available year-round. Both carrots and pumpkin are rich in vitamin A and potassium, essential nutrients for a growing brain.

1. Put the corn and coconut milk in a blender. Blend until smooth.

2. Add the steamed carrots to the mixture and purée until smooth.

3. Add the pumpkin and pulse to mix.

4. Strain through a cheesecloth, if desired, for a smoother mixture.

CHANGE IT UP: Add ½ teaspoon of pumpkin pie spice, cinnamon, or cumin to boost the flavor.

CHICKEN AND CARROTS

GLUTEN-FREE **NUT-FREE**

YIELDS 6 TO 9 SERVINGS

2 boneless, skinless chicken thighs, cubed

3 carrots, peeled and sliced

½ to ¾ cup low-sodium chicken or vegetable broth (or water)

½ teaspoon garlic powder

Pinch ground ginger

CHANGE IT UP: You can substitute squash or zucchini for the carrots. Expose your baby to some seasonings by adding a pinch of cinnamon, cumin, or rosemary.

Meat isn't often thought of as a first food, but as babies grow, they need iron and zinc. Both minerals are in chicken. Although you can use chicken breast for this recipe, using dark meat from a thigh will yield a smoother texture and higher iron levels. You can make this recipe in a rice cooker, a slow cooker, a pressure cooker, or a pot with a steamer insert.

1. Put the chicken and carrots in a steamer insert in a stockpot. Pour the broth into the pot, cover, and steam for 10 minutes.

2. Add the chicken and carrots to the broth along with the garlic and ginger, then purée by using a blender, a food processor, or an immersion blender with a tall cylinder container.

BABY-LED FEEDING TIP: Cut the chicken into strips rather than cubes and stop after step 1. Season with a sprinkling of garlic powder and serve. Chicken cubes can be a choking hazard as they are similar in size to a baby's esophagus and can get stuck easily. Strips will encourage your baby to develop good grip and learn to take appropriately sized bites.

BLACK BEAN, CORN, AND BROWN RICE INFANT PURÉE

GLUTEN-FREE **NUT-FREE** VEGAN

YIELDS 9 SERVINGS

½ cup sweet
corn, steamed

½ cup chopped
red bell pepper

Pinch cumin

1 teaspoon lime juice

2 cups cooked
black beans

½ cup Brown Rice
(page 30)

¼ cup low-sodium
vegetable broth

Corn is a starchy vegetable that is high in fiber, vitamins, and minerals. Black beans are a great vegetarian source of protein, iron, and folate. They make for great meals at all ages and are delicious with a side of Guacamole (page 161). Purée to a thicker texture for increased texture exposure.

1. Combine the corn, red bell pepper, cumin, and lime juice in a blender. Purée until smooth.

2. Add the black beans. Purée until smooth. The mixture will be thick.

3. Add the brown rice and vegetable broth. Purée to your desired texture. Serve warm.

CINNAMON APPLES AND PUMPKIN

GLUTEN-FREE **NUT-FREE** VEGAN

YIELDS 6 SERVINGS

1 tablespoon
lemon juice

12 ounces apples,
peeled and cored

10 ounces
canned pumpkin

1 teaspoon cinnamon

½ teaspoon nutmeg

This recipe is a perfect introduction to the fall season! Experiment with your favorite apples—some of mine are Honeycrisp, Golden Delicious, and Pink Lady. Since each apple has a different flavor, from super sweet to crisp and tart, this recipe introduces your little one to a range of flavors. The harvest spices can be intense, so start your baby with smaller amounts and work toward the full flavors. Pumpkin and apples are high-moisture foods, so you shouldn't need to add additional liquid.

1. Put the lemon juice and apples in a blender. Blend until smooth.

2. Add the pumpkin and pulse to mix.

3. Add the cinnamon and nutmeg and stir to fully incorporate.

4. Strain, if desired, for a smoother mixture.

GREEN BEANS, POTATOES, AND ZUCCHINI

GLUTEN-FREE **NUT-FREE** VEGAN

YIELDS 6 SERVINGS

¼ cup diced
Vidalia onion

2 teaspoons olive oil

1 white potato, peeled
and diced

½ cup trimmed and
chopped green beans

1 medium zucchini,
cut into large chunks

CHANGE IT UP:
Add a pinch of garlic
powder to boost
the flavor.

The green beans are the star of this purée. The mild flavors of potatoes and zucchini balance the strong flavor of fresh steamed green beans. Using the water that you steamed the zucchini and beans in retains the natural sodium and adds a touch of flavor.

1. In a pan over medium heat, sauté the onion in the olive oil for 3 minutes, or until translucent. Set aside.

2. Bring water to a boil in a medium pot, then add the potato and cook for 12 to 15 minutes, or until fork-tender. Set aside.

3. Discard the potato water, then add ¼ cup of clean water to the pot. Steam the green beans and zucchini for 7 minutes.

4. Allow all the ingredients to cool to room temperature.

5. Blend the onion, potato, green beans, and zucchini together until smooth in the water that remains from steaming the zucchini and beans.

6. Strain, if desired, for a smoother mixture.

COOKING TIP: Onions have a harsh flavor that is reduced when they are sautéed, but you can omit the onion if your baby has an aversion or allergy to it.

BABY-LED FEEDING TIP: Skip the onions, stop at step 4, add a pinch of garlic powder, and serve.

PEAR, KIWIFRUIT, AND SPINACH PURÉE

GLUTEN-FREE **NUT-FREE** VEGAN

YIELDS 6 SERVINGS

1 Bartlett pear, peeled, cored, and quartered

1 cup steamed sweet peas

1 cup spinach, stems trimmed

2 kiwifruits, peeled, quartered, and white pith removed from center

4 ounces coconut water, plus more if desired

Balancing the mild flavor of raw spinach with the sweet intensity of a pear gives your baby the opportunity to appreciate tasty foods that are decidedly green. Spinach grows low to the ground, so rinse it well from the leaves down to the stems, which are packed with vitamin A, potassium, and folate. For increased texture exposure, use a potato masher to smash the pears and kiwifruits, leaving these soft foods in very small chunks rather than puréeing them.

1. Place the pear, peas, spinach, and kiwifruits in a blender.

2. Blend and purée until smooth, adding a little coconut water at a time to achieve the desired consistency.

3. Strain, if desired, for a smoother texture.

CHERRY, APPLE, AND SWEET CORN YOGURT POPS

GLUTEN-FREE **NUT-FREE** **VEGETARIAN**

YIELDS 9 SERVINGS

1 cup sweet corn

1 apple, peeled and cored

1 cup cherries, pitted and stemmed

½ banana

6 ounces plain full-fat Greek yogurt

Mini pops are an amazing treat on a hot day. I love the Zoku mini pops mold for this recipe; it creates a great size and shape for exploring new foods. Thaw one pop in the refrigerator overnight for a protein-packed breakfast. A nondairy yogurt, like creamy cashew milk yogurt, is a good substitution if your baby has a dairy allergy. If you do not have a fine mesh sieve, you can use an old, clean T-shirt to line a colander.

1. In a saucepan over medium heat, steam the sweet corn for 3 to 5 minutes, then drain and let cool to room temperature.

2. Put the corn, apple, cherries, and banana in a blender. Purée until smooth.

3. Strain the mixture through a fine mesh sieve. Discard the remaining thick paste.

4. Stir in the yogurt and whisk until smooth.

5. Pour the mixture into an ice pop mold and freeze for at least 4 hours, up to overnight.

SPINACH, ZUCCHINI, AND QUINOA PURÉE

GLUTEN-FREE   NUT-FREE   VEGAN

YIELDS 6 SERVINGS

1 teaspoon olive oil

1 garlic clove, minced

1 medium zucchini, quartered

2 cups spinach, stems trimmed

6 ounces coconut cream

½ cup quinoa, steamed

1 ounce coconut milk, plus more if desired

This mild, creamy recipe is packed with green vegetables. The coconut cream makes this purée smooth and silky while reducing the strong flavor of the spinach.

1. Heat the olive oil in a skillet on medium heat. Sauté the garlic for 2 minutes. Remove from heat and transfer to a blender.

2. Add the zucchini, spinach, coconut cream, and quinoa to the blender and purée until smooth.

3. Add the coconut milk to achieve the desired thickness, adding more to make a thinner mixture.

4. Strain, if desired, for a smoother texture.

CHANGE IT UP: Add ¼ teaspoon of mild curry powder to kick up the flavor.

APPLE, MANGO, AND KALE PURÉE WITH CHIA SEEDS

`GLUTEN-FREE` `NUT-FREE` `VEGAN`

YIELDS 6 SERVINGS

1 apple, peeled, cored, and cut into chunks

1 mango, peeled, pitted, and cubed

1 pear, peeled, cored, and cut into chunks

1 cup kale, stems removed

1 tablespoon chia seeds

This recipe uses raw kale, which is rich in nutrients. As tempting as it is to buy bagged, diced kale, stick to the organic fresh kale on the stem. Kale stems can be chewy and bitter, so they should be removed. It takes more work to trim the stems from the bagged kale pieces than it does to trim them from a full leaf.

1. Put the apple, mango, pear, and kale in a blender.

2. Purée until smooth.

3. Strain the mixture through a fine mesh sieve, discarding any thick solids.

4. Add the chia seeds and stir to mix.

5. Cover the purée and let it sit for 20 minutes at room temperature before eating.

ROASTED SPAGHETTI SQUASH

GLUTEN-FREE **NUT-FREE** VEGAN

YIELDS 8 SERVINGS

1 tablespoon olive oil, plus more for greasing

1 spaghetti squash, halved

2 teaspoons cumin

2 teaspoons garlic powder

CHANGE IT UP: Try seasoning the squash with 1 tablespoon of Parmesan cheese or 2 teaspoons of cinnamon.

TO FREEZE: Tightly seal in a freezer-friendly container for up to 8 months.

Spaghetti squash is easy to cook and fun for kids of all ages. Watch your baby's face as you scrape the squash into noodles—soon your baby can help! To add some protein and make this a whole meal, drain and rinse a can of black beans and add the beans to the squash.

1. Preheat the oven to 400°F.

2. Rub the oil over the entire squash. Prepare a baking sheet by lining it with foil and coating it with oil. Place the squash on the baking sheet, cut-side down, and bake for about 40 minutes, until cooked through and soft.

3. Let the squash cool, then remove the seeds and strings.

4. Using two forks, shred the spaghetti squash to make noodles.

5. Sprinkle in the cumin and garlic powder and mix well.

TO REFRIGERATE: Wrap the squash in plastic or put it in a zip-top bag, tightly sealed, and store for up to 3 days.

PURÉE TIP: Simply purée the final product in a blender or food processor.

TOAST WITH NUT BUTTER

GLUTEN-FREE OPTION | **NUT-FREE OPTION** | VEGAN

YIELDS 2 SERVINGS

1 slice of bread (gluten-free bread optional)

Nut or seed butter

CHANGE IT UP:
Add a shake of cinnamon for an extra flavor burst.

It's important to introduce allergenic foods early, unless you're specifically advised otherwise. A great way to introduce nuts is with nut butters. You can try different types, like peanut, cashew, and almond. Sunflower seed or soy nut butter is an option if your doctor has advised to avoid peanuts or tree nuts.

1. Lightly toast the bread.

2. Thinly spread the nut butter on top of the toast.

3. Cut into triangles.

SAFETY TIP: Untoasted bread can be a choking hazard as soft bread turns into a dough ball in your baby's mouth. Bread that is overly toasted is difficult for them to manage. Aim for a golden color for the perfect toast.

ROASTED BROCCOLI

GLUTEN-FREE **NUT-FREE** VEGAN

YIELDS 5 SERVINGS

1 tablespoon olive
oil (plus extra for
greasing, optional)

2 garlic cloves, minced

Pinch kosher salt

3 cups broccoli florets

1 lemon wedge

CHANGE IT UP:
Increase the flavor
experience by adding
a pinch of onion
powder or black
pepper to the oil
mixture.

Broccoli's bright green color, its different textures, and the fact that it looks like little trees make it the perfect kids' food. Roasting cruciferous vegetables, like broccoli, cabbage, and Brussels sprouts, brings out a sweet undertone that makes them the perfect accompaniment to any main dish.

1. Preheat the oven to 425°F.

2. Prepare a baking sheet by lining it with parchment paper. If desired, lightly coat the baking sheet with olive oil.

3. In a small bowl, mix the olive oil with the garlic and salt.

4. Toss the broccoli in the oil mixture, then spread it out evenly on the baking sheet.

5. Bake for 10 to 12 minutes.

6. Squeeze the lemon juice over the broccoli just before serving.

TO REFRIGERATE: Store in a sealed container for up to 3 days.

PURÉE TIP: Blend the final product until slightly chunky. You may consider mixing this purée with mashed potatoes for a great texture.

BAKED SWEET POTATO FRIES

GLUTEN-FREE **NUT-FREE** VEGAN

YIELDS 8 SERVINGS

2 pounds sweet potatoes

1 tablespoon cornstarch (optional)

½ teaspoon kosher salt

2 tablespoons olive oil or melted butter, plus more for greasing

Pinch cinnamon

Sweet potatoes are versatile and delicious. They provide important fiber (particularly if the skin is left on), vitamin A, and vitamin C. Sweet potatoes also have a high antioxidant level that helps promote health and well-being. For younger babies, you'll want to cut the potatoes thicker or cook for less time so the fries are easy to chew and not crunchy.

1. Preheat the oven to 425°F.

2. Prepare a baking sheet by lightly coating it with olive oil.

3. Wash and scrub the sweet potatoes. Scrub them thoroughly if you're keeping the skin.

4. Cut the potatoes into sticks about ¼ inch wide and ¼ inch thick.

5. Place the fries into a large bowl or plastic bag.

6. If using cornstarch, toss the fries in cornstarch and salt, then spread them out on the prepared baking sheet in a single layer. Drizzle with olive oil, then sprinkle with cinnamon.

7. If not using cornstarch, toss the fries in olive oil, sprinkle with salt and cinnamon, and then spread them out on the prepared baking sheet in a single layer.

8. Bake for 20 minutes, then flip and bake for another 15 minutes.

TO FREEZE: These fries generally don't keep well in the refrigerator. Freeze them by placing the cooled fries in a single layer on a baking sheet. If you have more than one layer, place a sheet of parchment paper between the layers so the fries don't touch. Freeze for 1 hour, then remove and place in a sealed container for up to 6 months.

CHANGE IT UP: You can use the same recipe with carrots. Bake at 350°F for 12 minutes. Consider replacing cinnamon with Parmesan cheese or garlic for a different flavor experience.

COOKING TIP: If your fries get mushy, simply purée them and try again next time, cutting the fries thinner.

SAVORY PEA FRITTERS

GLUTEN-FREE OPTION **NUT-FREE** VEGETARIAN

YIELDS 7 SERVINGS

1 cup frozen peas

1 large egg

½ cup self-rising flour
(gluten-free flour
optional)

1½ tablespoons
shredded cheese, like
feta or Cheddar

1 tablespoon olive oil
or butter

CHANGE IT UP:
Replace some of the
peas with the same
amount of shredded
carrot or zucchini.

TO FREEZE: Wrap
the fritters individu-
ally and freeze for up
to 3 months.

Peas are a surprising source of protein, and their bright green color makes mealtime fun for babies. Serve these fritters, inspired by Healthy Little Foodies, with a dip, like Tzatziki (page 161) or Hummus (page 89), for additional nutrition.

1. In a saucepan, bring 3 cups of water to a boil. Add the peas and cook for 3 to 4 minutes. Drain and pat dry.

2. Add half of the peas, along with the egg, flour, and cheese, to a blender or food processor and blend until smooth.

3. Add the remaining peas to the blended mixture. Shape the mixture into fritters.

4. Heat the olive oil in a sauté pan over medium-high heat. Cook the fritters for about 2 minutes on each side, until slightly brown.

5. Let the fritters cool to room temperature or until slightly warm before serving.

TO REFRIGERATE: Store in an airtight container for up to 3 days.

COOKING TIPS: If your child isn't a fan of the chunky texture, you can blend all the peas at once. If you do not have self-rising flour, use all-purpose flour or all-purpose gluten-free flour and add ¾ teaspoon of baking powder and a pinch of salt.

PEANUT BUTTER COOKIES

GLUTEN-FREE **NUT-FREE OPTION** **VEGAN**

YIELDS 8 SERVINGS

1 (15.5-ounce) can chickpeas, drained and rinsed

3 teaspoons vanilla extract

¾ cup plus 2 tablespoons natural peanut butter or seed butter

⅓ cup maple syrup

1½ teaspoons baking powder

1 tablespoon light-tasting oil, such as light olive oil or avocado oil

CHANGE IT UP: For children over the age of two, you can add ½ cup of chocolate chips after blending but before rolling the dough into balls.

It can be difficult to know how to safely expose your baby to peanuts. This recipe is great for giving your child the benefit of safe and early exposure, which has been proven to help prevent the incidence of allergic reactions. These cookies are delicious and easy to grab. Use a food processor for this recipe since the dough is too thick for a traditional or immersion blender.

1. Preheat the oven to 350°F. Prepare a baking sheet by lining it with parchment paper or by lightly coating it with oil.

2. Blend the chickpeas, vanilla, peanut butter, maple syrup, baking powder, and oil together in a food processor.

3. Roll the dough into balls, about 1 inch in diameter.

4. Bake for 12 to 15 minutes.

5. Let cool and enjoy.

TO REFRIGERATE: Store in a sealed container for 3 to 4 days.

TO FREEZE: Store in a sealed container and freeze for up to 4 months.

NUTRITION TIP: You can add ½ cup of shelled sunflower seeds or finely chopped nuts for added nutrition and texture.

CARROT CUSTARD TARTS

GLUTEN-FREE OPTION | **NUT-FREE** | VEGETARIAN

YIELDS 12 SERVINGS

16 ounces jarred carrot purée

6 Medjool dates, pitted and soaked in warm water for at least 15 minutes

4 large eggs

1 cup all-purpose flour (gluten-free flour optional)

CHANGE IT UP: Use this recipe with many different vegetable purées, such as squash, pumpkin, or even broccoli, purée with seasoning to match: ½ teaspoon of cinnamon with squash, 1 teaspoon of pumpkin pie spice with pumpkin, or 1 teaspoon of garlic powder with broccoli.

Children of any age will love these delicious little tarts. Carrots are full of vibrant flavor and provide vitamin A for strong eyes, biotin for energy, and vitamin K for bone health.

1. Preheat the oven to 350°F. Line a muffin tin with paper or silicone liners.

2. Blend the carrot purée, dates, eggs, and flour together in a food processor or blender.

3. Fill each muffin cup three-quarters full.

4. Bake for 20 to 25 minutes, until the tarts puff slightly.

5. Remove from the oven and let cool. Tarts will reduce in size.

TO REFRIGERATE: Store in an airtight container for up to 4 days.

TO FREEZE: Store in an airtight container for up to 6 months.

COOKING TIP: You can use homemade carrot purée, but it may take 10 to 20 minutes longer in the oven depending on the moisture level. You'll know the tarts are done when they puff slightly and turn a golden color on top.

QUINOA PIZZA BITES

GLUTEN-FREE **NUT-FREE** **VEGETARIAN**

**YIELDS 12
SERVINGS**

1 tablespoon olive oil, plus extra for greasing

1 cup cooked quinoa

½ cup shredded cheese, plus
2 tablespoons

1 large egg

3 tablespoons low-sodium marinara or pizza sauce

¼ teaspoon garlic powder

CHANGE IT UP: To increase the flavor, add 2 to 3 teaspoons of dried Italian seasoning.

Quinoa is often overlooked as a baby food, but with baby-led feeding, it is versatile and appropriate for all ages. Quinoa is technically a seed and has a bit more protein than other grains.

1. Preheat the oven to 400°F. Prepare a mini-muffin pan by lightly coating each muffin cup with oil.

2. In a bowl, mix the olive oil, quinoa, ½ cup of shredded cheese, egg, marinara, and garlic powder.

3. Pour the mixture into the muffin cups, packing it down into each cup.

4. Bake for 12 minutes.

5. Remove from the oven and top with the remaining 2 tablespoons of cheese.

6. Bake for another 3 to 4 minutes, until the cheese begins to brown.

7. Remove from the oven and let cool.

TO REFRIGERATE: Store in a sealed container for up to a week.

TO FREEZE: Store in a sealed container for up to 3 months.

TWO-INGREDIENT PANCAKES

GLUTEN-FREE **NUT-FREE** VEGETARIAN

YIELDS 4 SERVINGS

2 large eggs

1 yellow banana, just ripe

⅓ teaspoon cinnamon (optional)

2 teaspoons olive oil or butter

CHANGE IT UP: Add a few blueberries and ¼ teaspoon of cinnamon.

These two-ingredient pancakes couldn't be easier. They are quick and tasty, and there are many ways to shake up the ingredients. Bananas are high in potassium and fiber, and the eggs provide protein and fat for a satisfying feeling. This dough is very thin, so make small pancakes to keep them from falling apart as you flip them.

1. Blend the eggs and banana (or mash the banana with a fork and then whisk with the eggs). Stir in the cinnamon, if using.

2. Heat the oil in a pan over medium heat. Using a tablespoon, drop the batter into the pan.

3. Cook until the edges of the pancakes begin to brown, then flip and cook for about 30 seconds longer.

4. Let cool and enjoy.

TO REFRIGERATE: Store in a sealed container for 1 to 2 days.

TO FREEZE: Let the pancakes cool completely, then store in an airtight container for up to 3 months.

MINI MEATLOAF

GLUTEN-FREE **NUT-FREE**

YIELDS 12 SERVINGS

1 tablespoon olive oil, plus more for greasing

½ onion, roughly chopped

1 small zucchini, roughly chopped

1 pound ground meat

1 large egg

¼ cup old-fashioned oats

TO REFRIGERATE: Keep in a sealed container for 3 to 4 days.

TO FREEZE: Keep in an airtight container for up to 5 months.

This recipe is great for the whole family! Meat provides iron and zinc, which are among the very few nutrients not supplied by breast milk, though many formulas are fortified. When serving mini muffins, you can give them to your baby without cutting them up. When serving full-size meatloaf muffins, cut one into quarters to make it easier for the baby to handle.

1. Preheat the oven to 350°F.

2. Prepare a mini-muffin pan by lightly coating each muffin cup with olive oil.

3. In a blender or food processor, blend the onion and zucchini until smooth. Transfer to a large bowl.

4. Add the meat, egg, oats, and oil. Use a potato masher to combine.

5. Using your hands or a tablespoon, scoop about 1 tablespoon of the mixture into each muffin well.

6. Bake for about 20 minutes, until the edges begin to brown and come away from the sides and the internal temperature reaches 165°F. If you are making full-size muffins, bake for an additional 10 minutes.

COOKING TIP: If you are using white meat ground turkey, the muffins may come out a bit dry, so consider adding some beef and making a double batch.

CHANGE IT UP: Boost the flavor by adding some of these ingredients:
- 2 garlic cloves, minced, blended with the onion and zucchini
- 2 teaspoons of oregano
- 2 teaspoons of Italian seasoning

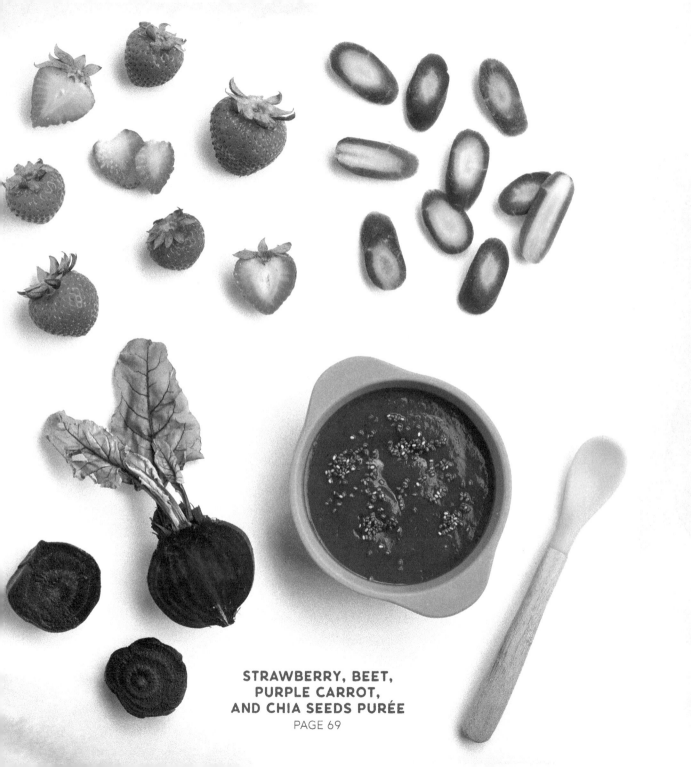

**STRAWBERRY, BEET,
PURPLE CARROT,
AND CHIA SEEDS PURÉE**
PAGE 69

3

STAGE TWO GUIDE AND RECIPES

At this stage, things get really fun. Your baby starts to develop a distinct personality and reacts when you use their name. At this point, they see food as connection with the caregiver—an opportunity for valuable interaction. They find the colors, smells, and flavors of different foods fascinating.

RECURSIVE

BABY AT THIS STAGE

Your baby is exploring boundaries and going wherever curiosity leads. And food is a fun way to feed that curiosity!

DEVELOPMENTAL SKILLS

At this point, your baby is becoming more independent. Maybe they have started to roll, scoot, or crawl. You may notice some teeth starting to come in, which can cause increased drooling and fussiness. Your baby is likely still grasping objects with a full fist but is working toward that pincer grasp. And this is prime time for curiosity, which you can and should use to introduce all kinds of new food experiences.

NUTRITIONAL NEEDS

Your baby's nutritional needs have increased overall since the six-month mark, but the concepts remain the same. Breast milk or formula is still the primary source of nutrition and should be offered on demand, before solid food. Your baby will be drinking six to eight ounces, six times per day, but babies, just like adults, have days when they are more or less hungry. Follow your baby's hunger and fullness cues to know how much to provide.

Whether you've chosen the purée route, baby-led feeding, or a combination of the two, eating solid food remains an activity and not the main source for your baby's nutrition. As discussed in chapter 1, however, your baby does require iron, zinc, and vitamin D.

WHAT TO INTRODUCE

Although baby cereal is a common first food in North America, that isn't the case everywhere. Mark your baby's gustatory passport or keep it simple.

FOODS AND FLAVORS

There are no rules regarding which flavors to introduce or when. In fact, reading articles about what babies eat around the world might help you confidently introduce a powerful flavor. In China, it's common to give babies seaweed, fish, and smashed eggplant. In Mexico, it's common to sprinkle chili powder and squeeze lime juice onto foods at an early age.

Remember, babies' taste buds are very sensitive and can pick up subtle flavors. Simple treats such as raspberries with yogurt, sourdough toast with butter, or oatmeal with smashed fruit or veggie purée will be a cause for celebration.

TOOLS AND UTENSILS

Continue to use the same tools you've been using, although you can try different brands if you're so inclined. Your baby will continue to progress in using utensils, but don't be surprised if their favorite utensil continues to be a cute little fist. Utensil use is a skill that develops slowly.

TYPICAL MEALS AND SCHEDULE

Mealtime remains a valuable activity at six to eight months of age. Continue using the size of your baby's fist as a reference for serving size, keeping in mind that they may be interested in more food, or less, from meal to meal. Keeping serving sizes small ensures a positive experience as your baby is less likely to get overwhelmed and overstimulated by too much food.

A typical meal can start to progress in complexity. If you started with single-item purées, you can provide more depth of flavor and texture. For example, where you may have given your baby a banana, you might add some yogurt on the side. And if you chose to hit the ground running with more complex dishes, that's great, too.

Your baby continues the eat, sleep, and play pattern, being awake for no more than two to two and a half hours between naps. Different family dynamics will call for different schedules, and this one does not need to be followed to the minute. For additional scheduling options, please see Resources (page 189).

TASTY TEETHER FOODS

Teething can start at different times for different babies. Did you know that one in every 2,000 babies is actually born with teeth? Babies react to teething in different ways; some drool and become fussy, while others show no outward signs and then suddenly teeth appear.

6:00 A.M.	Wake and feed (breast milk or formula)
7:45 A.M.	Solid food breakfast
8:00 A.M.	Nap (45 to 60 minutes or more)
9:30 A.M.	Wake and feed (breast milk or formula)
10:00 A.M.	Snack option #1
11:30 A.M.	Nap (1½ to 2 hours or more)
2:00 P.M.	Wake and feed (breast milk or formula)
2:30 P.M.	Snack option #2
3:30 P.M.	Nap (20 to 60 minutes)
5:00 P.M.	Solid food dinner
5:30 P.M.	Begin bedtime routine
6:00 P.M.	Breast milk or formula, then to bed

If your baby is irritable during this time, they may find comfort in chewing on a washcloth that has been soaked in water and frozen. You can also try mesh teethers filled with frozen peas or frozen pineapple chunks. Some babies dislike the cold sensation and prefer a teething biscuit or even a large piece of raw broccoli. These are not meals or snacks, as the baby is simply using them for teething, but they do serve a creative nutritional purpose. These foods give valuable exposure to your baby, which means that when you do serve them on a plate at mealtime, they are more likely to be accepted.

Other teething foods can be given as a snack or part of a meal, serving a dual purpose. Bamba is a widely available puffed peanut snack. It is easy to grab and grip, it's tasty, and it provides that early peanut exposure mentioned in the Allergies section in chapter 1.

Many times, a baby will get an oral rash from drooling or a diaper rash during teething. If this is happening, avoid acidic foods, such as citrus, pineapple, or tomato products, which can irritate a baby's sensitive skin.

COMMON CHALLENGES

YOUR BABY DOESN'T SEEM INTERESTED IN FOOD: It's important to feed responsively. Here are some guidelines to follow:

* Place your baby in a comfortable seat that supports their feet and back.

* Do not rush your baby or take food away before they are finished.

* Allow your baby space to explore by not being too close or too excited.

Sometimes, your baby will make a funny face or give a seemingly negative reaction when introduced to a food. This reaction is not necessarily a rejection. If you leave the food there, the baby may or may not try it again. Sometimes it takes 15 to 20 exposures before your baby is willing to taste the food again. Maintain a zero-pressure environment at the table, and your baby will feel confident and supported enough to be adventurous.

YOUR BABY KEEPS TRYING TO GRAB THE SPOON: Sometimes a feeding method chooses us. If you chose to start with purées and it isn't going well, consider baby-led feeding. Babies at this stage are so curious and interested in independence. Let your baby take the lead. Load up the spoon and place it on the tray for them to grab or give them a piece of buttered toast or some Baked Sweet Potato Fries (page 44).

YOUR BABY PREFERS SOLID FOOD OVER THE BREAST OR BOTTLE: First, check your schedule. The breast or bottle should be given before solid food. Your baby should have no more than two or three solid meals per day at this point, and those are activities, not meaningful nutrition. Ensure there is no pressure with the bottle, breast, or solid food meals. And finally, be sure that the solid food meals are simple with no added sugars. You may consider the possibility of oral-motor challenges, which make breastfeeding or bottle-feeding difficult and solid food feeding easier. A lip or tongue tie or a history of reflux may cause your baby to feel more comfortable with solid foods than with the breast or bottle. Speak to your pediatrician or lactation consultant about these concerns. (See Resources on page 190 for how to connect to an international board-certified lactation consultant.) Many pediatric dentists can identify these obstacles as well, and now is an appropriate time to bring your baby for their first dental checkup.

COTTAGE CHEESE WITH MIX-INS

GLUTEN-FREE **NUT-FREE** **VEGETARIAN**

YIELDS 1 SERVING

⅓ cup cottage cheese (no salt added)

Soft fruit, such as berries, pears, or peeled stone fruits

NUTRITION TIP:
Add 1 teaspoon of ground flax meal for added fat and fiber.

Cottage cheese is a fun base for a purée because it comes in different textures: small curd, large curd, and blended for a smooth effect. Check the ingredient list to be sure there is no added salt, and choose one made with whole milk. Fat is important for your baby's developing brain, so stick with whole-milk dairy options as much as possible, at least for the first two years. If the baby doesn't like it at first, let them try it again a few days later with a different add-in or a different texture.

1. Add the cottage cheese to your baby's bowl.

2. In a separate small bowl, mash the fruit with a fork.

3. Add the mashed fruit to cottage cheese—you may stir, blend, or leave it on top for different experiences.

STORAGE TIPS FOR ALL PURÉES:

TO REFRIGERATE: Store in a sealed container in the refrigerator for up to 5 days.

TO FREEZE: Portion into ice cube trays or a silicone baby food freezer tray. Freeze, then pop the cubes out and store in an airtight container for up to 3 months, removing each portion as needed. Defrost in one of three different ways:

- Let the purée thaw overnight in the fridge.
- Place sealed frozen bags of purées in a warm water bath until thawed.
- Place frozen baby food in a microwave-safe dish and use the defrost function on your microwave to thaw. Stir frequently and be sure that the food is the appropriate temperature prior to serving.

TO SERVE: Serve thawed baby food within 48 hours of defrosting. Discard any food that remains beyond that time.

SWEET POTATO, APPLE, AND LENTIL PURÉE

GLUTEN-FREE **NUT-FREE** VEGAN

YIELDS 4 SERVINGS

1 cup water or low-sodium chicken or vegetable broth

½ cup dry green, yellow, or red lentils, rinsed

1 sweet potato, peeled and cut into chunks

2 apples, peeled, cored, and cut into chunks

¼ teaspoon cinnamon

CHANGE IT UP:
Consider adding or substituting a small shake of nutmeg or a pinch of ground ginger.

Lentils are often overlooked when considering purées. But they are a nutrition powerhouse, providing protein, vitamins, antioxidants, fiber, and iron. Lentils also cook easily and blend so nicely.

1. In a saucepan, bring the water to a boil and add the lentils.

2. Cover the pot and turn the heat down to let the lentils simmer for 30 to 40 minutes, until all the liquid is absorbed and the lentils are soft.

3. In another pot (or rice cooker), insert a steamer tray and add a little water.

4. Bring the water to a boil, then add the sweet potato and apples. Steam for 10 minutes, or until cooked through and soft.

5. Blend the lentils, sweet potato, apples, and cinnamon with a blender or food processor until smooth.

COOKING TIP: You may substitute a hard squash, such as butternut or acorn, for the sweet potato.

APPLE AND RASPBERRY PURÉE

GLUTEN-FREE NUT-FREE VEGAN

YIELDS 1 TO 2 SERVINGS

1 tablespoon olive oil or unsalted butter

1 apple, peeled, cored, and chopped into thumb-size chunks

Pinch cinnamon (optional)

¼ cup raspberries

COOKING TIP: Substitute pears for the apples and decrease cooking time to about 20 minutes.

Roasting fruits and veggies can bring out a delicious caramel taste that appeals to taste buds of all ages. These roasted apples pair nicely with smashed raspberry and provide your baby with a colorful meal experience.

1. Preheat the oven to 350°F.

2. Prepare a baking sheet by lining it with foil and coating it lightly with the olive oil or butter.

3. Lay the apple chunks in a single layer on the prepared baking sheet. Lightly dust with cinnamon, if using.

4. Bake for 25 to 30 minutes, or until soft.

5. Soak the raspberries in a separate bowl of water for a few minutes, then drain.

6. Let the apples cool, then add them to the raspberries. Blend or mash together.

BABY-LED FEEDING TIP: Serve apple chunks as they are and cut the raspberries in half.

BEEF AND PUMPKIN PURÉE

GLUTEN-FREE **NUT-FREE**

YIELDS 6 TO 8 SERVINGS

8 ounces chuck beef, trimmed and chopped

1 cup chopped pumpkin or 1 (15-ounce) can pumpkin purée

1 white or sweet potato, peeled and chopped

1 bay leaf

COOKING TIP: You may substitute the pumpkin with butternut or acorn squash.

When puréeing meat, pair it with a creamy vegetable to help offset its dry texture. This recipe features fresh pumpkin, which makes it perfect for the fall months. Pumpkin is a great source of vitamin K, which is important for bone growth.

1. Put the beef, chopped pumpkin, potato, and bay leaf in a saucepan and cover with water. If using pumpkin purée, reserve it to add later.

2. Cover the pot and bring to a boil, then simmer for about 35 minutes. Add water as needed.

3. Remove the meat and vegetables from the pot but reserve the cooking liquid. Discard the bay leaf.

4. Blend all the ingredients together. (If you're using pumpkin purée, add it now.) Add some cooking liquid a little at a time until the desired texture is reached.

BABY-LED FEEDING TIP: Cut the beef into long strips rather than chunks. The strip should fit in your baby's palmar grasp with a bit of steak sticking out of the top of their fist. Serve after completing step 3.

CHICKEN AND MANGO PURÉE

GLUTEN-FREE **NUT-FREE**

YIELDS 12 SERVINGS

1 tablespoon olive oil

2 boneless, skinless chicken thighs

1 mango, peeled, pitted, and chopped

4 carrots, peeled and sliced

1 cup low-sodium chicken or vegetable broth

CHANGE IT UP: To make this an international voyage, try rubbing the chicken with ½ teaspoon of mild curry powder before cooking.

Mango is a flavorful fruit with a creamy texture that pairs perfectly with puréed chicken. The play of sweet and savory in this dish will be a party in your baby's mouth. Mangos are very high in vitamin C and provide a great boost of vitamin A for eye health and folate for healthy growth and development. Serving this dish with Brown Rice (page 30) will make this a satisfying meal.

1. Preheat the oven to 350°F. Prepare a baking sheet by coating it lightly with the olive oil.

2. Place the chicken, mango, and carrots on the foil, then wrap them in the foil like a package, sealing all edges.

3. Bake for 30 to 45 minutes, until the internal temperature of the chicken reaches 165°F.

4. Let the foods cool slightly, then blend them, slowly adding the broth until the desired texture has been reached.

BABY-LED FEEDING TIP: Stop at step 3 and cut the chicken into strips long enough to stick out of the top of your baby's fist.

SPINACH, PUMPKIN, AND CHICKPEAS

GLUTEN-FREE **NUT-FREE** VEGAN

YIELDS 6 SERVINGS

½ cup water

¼ cup old-fashioned oats

1 cup canned chickpeas, drained and rinsed

1 cup spinach, stems trimmed

½ cup broccoli florets, steamed

8 ounces low-sodium vegetable broth

½ cup canned pumpkin

½ teaspoon coriander

The pumpkin in this recipe adds a subtly sweet flavor to an otherwise savory purée. Combining it with chickpeas, which provide a protein punch, and oats gives this recipe a thick consistency, which is perfect as your baby grows into eating more solid foods. This recipe freezes well.

1. In a saucepan, bring the water to a boil.

2. Add the oats to the water and simmer for 5 minutes over low heat.

3. Combine the chickpeas, spinach, broccoli, and vegetable broth in a blender. Pulse into small chunks.

4. Add the oats, pumpkin, and coriander to the blender mixture and pulse until just mixed.

CARROT, SWEET POTATO, AND BROWN RICE

GLUTEN-FREE **NUT-FREE** VEGAN

YIELDS 6 SERVINGS

1 sweet potato, peeled and diced

2 large carrots, peeled and diced

¾-inch piece fresh ginger, grated

½ cup Brown Rice (page 30)

This recipe produces a beautifully orange food. Pulsing the carrots and sweet potatoes to a thick, chunky texture rather than a purée allows your baby to experience the texture of their foods. The brown rice nicely rounds out the consistency for an easy and versatile purée.

1. Boil the sweet potato and carrots for 7 to 10 minutes, or until fork-tender.

2. Allow the foods to cool to room temperature.

3. Pulse the sweet potato, carrots, ginger, and brown rice in a blender until the mixture is in small chunks.

BABY-LED FEEDING TIP: Stop after step 2, add a pinch of cinnamon or cumin, and serve.

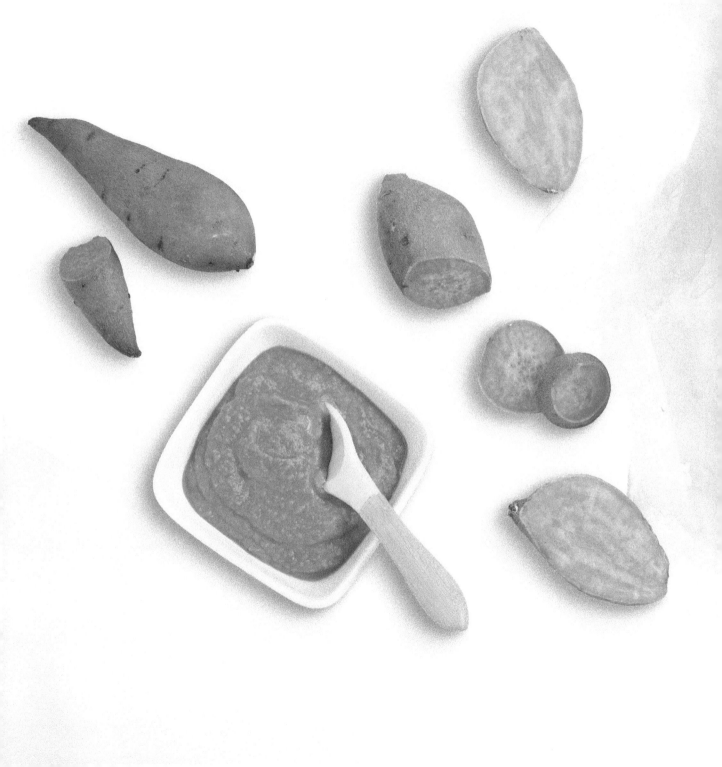

ROASTED PUMPKIN AND COCONUT RICE

GLUTEN-FREE **NUT-FREE** VEGAN

YIELDS 14 SERVINGS

1 Amish Pie pumpkin

1 tablespoon olive oil

½-inch piece ginger, peeled

4 ounces coconut water

1½ cups mango chunks

4 ounces full-fat canned coconut milk

½ cup Brown Rice (page 30)

Canned pumpkin is commercially available, but roasting your own adds a depth of flavor. The pairing of sweet foods with coconut milk enhances the flavors with a creamy texture. Add mango and something truly delicious emerges.

1. Preheat the oven to 350°F.

2. Cut the pumpkin into quarters, removing the seeds and pith. Rub the olive oil on the skin.

3. Line a shallow baking dish with parchment paper. Place the pumpkin skin-side up in the dish and roast for 20 minutes. Allow to cool completely.

4. Gently peel away the pumpkin's skin and discard.

5. Place 1 cup of roasted pumpkin, ginger, coconut water, and mango in a blender and purée until smooth.

6. In a bowl, mix the purée and coconut milk. Add the brown rice, mixing well.

7. Mash with a fork for smaller bites and serve.

BABY-LED FEEDING TIP: Instead of mashing the mixture, let your baby eat it with a spoon.

STRAWBERRY, BEET, PURPLE CARROT, AND CHIA SEEDS

GLUTEN-FREE **NUT-FREE** VEGAN

YIELDS 6 SERVINGS

1 beet

2 purple carrots, peeled and quartered

1 kiwifruit, peeled, quartered, and white pith removed from center

4 ounces pear nectar

10 strawberries, hulled and cut into bite-size chunks

1 tablespoon chia seeds

Purple carrots are great for both their color and their nutrients. They are deliciously sweet compared to their orange counterparts, although either can be used in this recipe. Beets enhance the sweetness of this dish, while strawberries add both color and a touch of tartness to balance the natural sugars. Experiment with different varieties of beets for different flavors. The chia seeds also make this recipe helpful if your baby is constipated.

1. Preheat the oven to 350°F.

2. Cut off the top of the beet, then cut the beet in half and poke each side with a fork.

3. Line a baking sheet with parchment paper. Place the beet on the prepared baking sheet and bake for 25 minutes, until fork-tender.

4. Let the beet cool to room temperature, then remove its tough outer skin. Cut into bite-size chunks.

5. Steam the carrots in a pot with shallow water until tender. Drain.

6. Put the kiwifruit, beet, purple carrots, pear nectar, and strawberries in a blender. Pulse until smooth.

7. Place the purée in a bowl, sprinkle with the chia seeds, and stir well to mix.

8. Cool to room temperature for 20 minutes before serving.

TROPICAL FRUITS MASH-UP

GLUTEN-FREE **NUT-FREE** VEGAN

YIELDS 6 SERVINGS

1 banana (red, if available)

2 ounces guava nectar

4 ounces pineapple nectar

8 ounces cubed mango, diced

1 pear, peeled, cored, and diced

2 apples, peeled, cored, and diced

Deliciously sweet, this recipe is only missing a hammock and ocean breeze. The smaller bite-size chunks make this purée a great starting point for your baby to begin feeding themselves. Alternatively, this recipe makes great frozen pops if you completely purée it. Portion the purée into your favorite mold and freeze for 4 to 6 hours or overnight.

1. Place the banana, guava nectar, and pineapple nectar in a blender.

2. Purée until smooth.

3. Add the purée to the diced mango, pear, and apples and mix well.

CHANGE IT UP: If your child is experiencing a diaper rash, skip the pineapple nectar.

APPLE-CINNAMON OATMEAL FINGERS

GLUTEN-FREE **NUT-FREE** VEGETARIAN VEGAN OPTION

YIELDS 6 TO 8 SERVINGS

4 tablespoons old-fashioned oats

2 tablespoons milk (milk alternative for vegan option)

2 tablespoons applesauce

1 tablespoon peeled and grated apple

½ teaspoon cinnamon

TO REFRIGERATE: Store in a sealed container for up to 3 days.

Oatmeal is filling and versatile. These oatmeal fingers, inspired by Healthy Little Foodies, travel well and are easily accepted by tiny taste buds. This recipe is mild and will appeal more to littles than to adults as babies pick up on subtle flavors that we often miss as we get older.

1. In a medium bowl, mix the oats, milk, and applesauce. Soak until the oats are mushy.

2. Stir in the grated apple and cinnamon.

3. Using the back of a spoon, press the mixture into a 9-by-13-inch baking dish.

4. Microwave on high for 2 minutes.

5. Cut into fingers while the food is hot, then let it cool to room temperature before serving.

TO FREEZE: Store in an airtight container for up to 3 months.

CHANGE IT UP: For a new flavor exposure, add a pinch of nutmeg. For added sweetness, mix in 4 to 5 chopped raisins or dried cranberries. These are not a choking hazard as cooking changes their texture, making them softer and easier to chew and swallow.

BAKED BROCCOLI BITES

GLUTEN-FREE OPTION **NUT-FREE** **VEGETARIAN** **VEGAN OPTION**

YIELDS 15 BITES

1 tablespoon olive oil (optional)

2 cups broccoli florets

1 large egg (flax egg for vegan option)

¼ cup grated Parmesan cheese (3 tablespoons nutritional yeast for vegan option)

½ cup panko bread crumbs (gluten-free bread crumbs optional)

1 teaspoon dried oregano

1 teaspoon garlic powder

CHANGE IT UP:
Consider adding 2 tablespoons of sun-dried tomatoes in oil (after patting them dry) and/or 1 teaspoon of Italian seasoning.

Inspired by *Pickled Plum*, these baked broccoli bites are the perfect size for little hands. Consider serving them with Hummus (page 89) or Tzatziki (page 161). Exposing your baby to broccoli in different forms during this golden window when everything is new and fun can help prevent food fear as your baby grows and becomes more hesitant with unfamiliar foods. If you are using leftover stems from another recipe, such as the Cauliflower Popcorn (page 75), replace up to a cup of the broccoli florets with shredded broccoli or cauliflower stems.

1. Preheat the oven to 375°F.

2. Line a baking sheet with foil or parchment paper. If using foil, lightly coat it with the olive oil.

3. Fill a large pot with water and blanch the broccoli by boiling it for 3 minutes. Drain and pat dry.

4. Place the broccoli in a food processor and pulse until finely chopped. Transfer to a large mixing bowl.

5. Add the egg, cheese, bread crumbs, oregano, and garlic powder to the bowl with the broccoli and mix thoroughly.

6. Using 2 tablespoons of the mixture, make tater tot–shaped bites with your hands and place on the prepared baking sheet.

7. Bake 20 to 25 minutes, until brown and crispy. Cool and serve.

TO REFRIGERATE: Store in a sealed container for up to 3 days.

TO FREEZE: Store in an airtight container for up to 3 months.

PASTA AND VEGGIEFUL SAUCE

GLUTEN-FREE OPTION **NUT-FREE** VEGAN

YIELDS 12
SERVINGS

1 tablespoon olive oil

4 ounces
(about 1 cup)
mushrooms, sliced

1 (26-ounce)
jar low-sodium
marinara sauce

6 ounces
butternut squash,
chopped small

1 medium
zucchini, chopped

12 ounces rotini or
other pasta (gluten-
free pasta optional),
cooked according to
package instructions

TO FREEZE: Store
in an airtight con-
tainer (such as a jar or
freezer bag) for up to
5 months.

Soups and sauces are a great way to provide a major veggie boost. To expose your little one to recognizable veggies, add some roasted or steamed whole vegetables to your dinner as well. This recipe is very forgiving—you can go a bit over or under on ingredients, and it will work just fine. This recipe makes a lot of sauce, so consider using the leftover sauce for Flatbread Pizza (page 136) or as a dip for the Baked Broccoli Bites (page 72)!

1. Heat the olive oil in a large saucepan. Add the mushrooms and sauté for about 8 minutes, or until the mushrooms are soft and reduced in size.

2. Warm the marinara in a saucepan over medium heat.

3. Add the mushrooms, butternut squash, and zucchini to the marinara and bring to a simmer. Simmer for 30 minutes.

4. Remove the sauce from heat. Using an immersion blender, blend the sauce to your desired consistency.

5. Add the sauce to the prepared pasta, then pour the extra sauce into jars while it's still hot. Allow to cool before storing.

TO REFRIGERATE: Store in a tightly sealed container for up to 5 days.

COOKING TIP: Even at this young age, babies can start to get involved in the kitchen. Show your baby how to add veggies to the pasta sauce base. There is a twofold benefit: awesome bonding time and exposure to more veggies as they're added to the pot!

RICOTTA PANCAKES

GLUTEN-FREE OPTION **NUT-FREE** VEGETARIAN

YIELDS 6 TO 8 PANCAKES

3 large eggs

1 cup ricotta cheese

1 teaspoon vanilla extract

2 tablespoons maple syrup

½ cup all-purpose flour (gluten-free flour optional)

1 teaspoon baking powder

¼ teaspoon kosher salt

Butter, oil, or nonstick cooking spray

CHANGE IT UP: Add some extra flavor with ½ teaspoon of lemon zest or a pinch of ground ginger.

These ricotta pancakes are wonderful for kids going through a selective phase. Ricotta has a natural sweetness and a smooth texture that lends itself very well to pancakes. These pancakes are high in protein and provide the calcium and fat so important for growth and development. Consider doubling or tripling the recipe and freezing the extra pancakes for later—leftovers are great for a quick breakfast or a snack on the go!

1. Mix the eggs, ricotta cheese, vanilla, and maple syrup together in a medium mixing bowl.

2. Add the flour, baking powder, and salt to the wet ingredients and whisk until just combined, being careful to avoid overmixing.

3. Heat a pat of butter in a large sauté pan or griddle over medium heat (if you have an electric griddle, heat to 300°F).

4. Using a ¼-cup measuring cup, scoop the batter onto the heated pan or griddle. Cook for 2 to 3 minutes on each side, or until golden.

TO REFRIGERATE: Leftover pancakes can be stored in an airtight container and kept in the refrigerator for 3 to 4 days.

TO FREEZE: Store in an airtight container and freeze for up to 4 months.

CAULIFLOWER POPCORN

GLUTEN-FREE **NUT-FREE** VEGAN

YIELDS 8 SERVINGS

¼ cup olive oil, plus
1 tablespoon

1 head cauliflower

1 teaspoon
kosher salt

½ teaspoon
garlic powder

½ teaspoon
onion powder

COOKING TIP: The longer these are cooked, the sweeter and crunchier they get. They can be cooked for up to an hour, depending on how large your pieces are.

Traditional popcorn is a choking hazard and should be avoided until four years of age, but this cauliflower popcorn is a delicious alternative to the popular snack, and it's perfect for baby-led feeding! Cauliflower is high in vitamin C to help support immunity and vitamin B6 for brain development.

1. Preheat the oven to 400°F. Prepare a baking sheet by lining it with foil and lightly coating with 1 tablespoon of olive oil or by lining it with parchment paper.

2. Cut the cauliflower into florets (the size of popped popcorn) and reserve the core and stems for Baked Broccoli Bites (page 72).

3. Toss the florets with the remaining ¼ cup of olive oil, salt, garlic powder, and onion powder.

4. Lay the florets in a single layer on the baking sheet and bake for 20 minutes, then flip and bake for another 20 minutes, or until they're golden on the outside and soft through the inside.

5. Let cool and serve.

TO REFRIGERATE: Store in a sealed container for up to 3 days. The florets may lose their crunch, but they will still be delicious.

CHANGE IT UP: For additional flavor, consider adding 1 teaspoon of mild curry powder or 1 to 2 teaspoons of nutritional yeast.

PURÉE TIP: After step 5, blend with low-sodium chicken or vegetable broth until you reach the desired texture.

CHOCOLATE BLOOMIES

NUT-FREE VEGETARIAN VEGAN OPTION

YIELDS 12 MUFFINS

6 dates, pitted and soaked in warm water

1 cup canned squash or pumpkin purée

¼ cup coconut oil

½ cup carrot juice, room temperature

1 large egg (flax egg for vegan option)

½ teaspoon vanilla extract

¾ cup whole-wheat flour

¾ cup oat flour

½ cup cocoa powder

1 teaspoon baking soda

¼ teaspoon salt

½ teaspoon cinnamon

1½ cups shredded zucchini

TO STORE: Store at room temperature for 3 to 5 days.

Loaded with natural sweetness, moisture, and potassium, this decadent recipe combines nutritious squash with chocolate. Balanced with zucchini and sweetened with fiber-rich dates, these bloomies are irresistible. I dare you to eat only one. Vegetarian and dairy-free, they are sure to be a playdate favorite.

1. Preheat the oven to 350°F. Prepare a muffin tin with paper liners or cooking oil.

2. Combine the dates, squash, coconut oil, carrot juice, egg, and vanilla in a blender and purée until smooth.

3. In a separate bowl, mix the whole-wheat flour, oat flour, cocoa powder, baking soda, salt, and cinnamon.

4. Add the wet ingredients to the dry mixture and mix until just combined.

5. Fold in the zucchini and mix to incorporate.

6. Bake for 15 to 20 minutes, until a toothpick inserted in the middle comes out clean.

7. Allow the bloomies to cool on a wire rack before serving.

TO REFRIGERATE: Store in a sealed container for 4 to 5 days.

TO FREEZE: Store in an airtight container for up to 5 months.

COOKING TIPS: Make your own oat flour by blending oats in a food processor. For this recipe, it's best to use shredded zucchini. You can purée the zucchini in step 2, but that will result in a more fudgy, undercooked-tasting product.

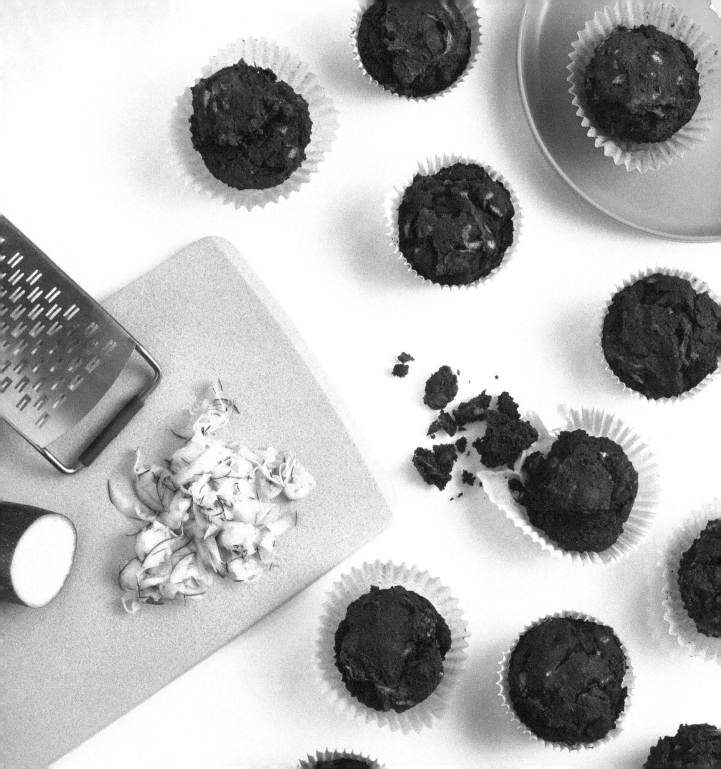

FRENCH TOAST STICKS

GLUTEN-FREE OPTION **NUT-FREE** VEGETARIAN

YIELDS 6 SERVINGS

2 large eggs

¼ cup milk or milk alternative

Butter, olive oil, or olive oil cooking spray (optional)

2 slices bread (gluten-free bread optional)

¼ teaspoon cinnamon

CHANGE IT UP:
You can increase the flavor profile by adding seasoning to the egg-and-milk mixture before soaking the bread. Consider adding ½ teaspoon of vanilla extract, ½ teaspoon of orange zest, or a pinch of freshly grated ginger.

Tasty French toast is wonderful at all ages. These French toast sticks are the perfect size for a baby's little fist and are high in fiber and protein. Most importantly, this is a food that parents and their baby can appreciate together.

1. In a medium bowl, beat the eggs, then add the milk and stir.

2. Heat a pan over medium heat and coat it with butter or olive oil. If using an electric griddle, heat to 300°F. No oil or butter is needed.

3. Cut each slice of bread into 3 long sticks and soak in the egg-and-milk mixture. If you are using dense bread, such as a sprouted whole-wheat version, poke the bread with a fork to allow the bread to fully absorb the liquid.

4. Lightly shake the cinnamon on top.

5. Place the French toast sticks in the pan. Cook for 2 to 3 minutes on each side, or until golden brown.

6. Serve warm.

TO REFRIGERATE: Store in a sealed container for up to 3 days.

TO FREEZE: Wrap with foil and store in an airtight container for up to 1 month.

ROASTED CARROTS

GLUTEN-FREE **NUT-FREE** VEGAN

YIELDS 6 TO 7 SERVINGS

Olive oil, butter, or olive oil cooking spray

3 carrots, peeled and cut into sticks

Pinch kosher salt

Pinch cinnamon

TO REFRIGERATE: Store in a sealed container for up to 3 days.

TO FREEZE: Wrap the carrots tightly with foil, then store in an airtight container for up to a month.

PURÉE TIP: After step 5, blend with low-sodium broth, formula, or expressed breast milk to achieve the desired texture.

Carrots are great to keep around the house. They can be used as teethers when raw, baked and combined with baked or puréed apples or oatmeal, and roasted for easy pickup by little hands. Carrots are naturally sweet, and, best of all, they pair well with many dishes and can be enjoyed by the whole family. For baby-led feeding, it's safer to serve these as sticks rather than cubes.

1. Preheat the oven to 425°F.

2. Line a baking sheet with parchment paper or foil. If using foil, coat it generously with olive oil or butter.

3. Lay the carrots in a single layer on the baking sheet, spray with olive oil, and sprinkle with salt and cinnamon.

4. Bake until golden brown, 20 to 25 minutes.

COOKING TIP: A longer cooking time will result in a sweeter and crispier carrot. You can experiment with this recipe to get the result you prefer.

CHANGE IT UP: You can increase the flavor exposure by adding some of these ingredients:
- ¼ to ½ teaspoon of garlic powder
- ¼ to ½ teaspoon of cumin
- Pinch of freshly grated ginger
- Sprinkling of Parmesan cheese

PARMESAN ROASTED ZUCCHINI

GLUTEN-FREE **NUT-FREE** VEGETARIAN

**YIELDS 12
SERVINGS**

**Olive oil cooking spray
(optional)**

**½ cup grated
Parmesan cheese**

**½ teaspoon
garlic powder**

**3 medium zucchini,
cut lengthwise
into wedges**

2 tablespoons olive oil

TO REFRIGERATE:
Store in a sealed container for up to 3 days.
The zucchini will lose
its crunch.

Zucchini is a fun and versatile vegetable that is actually a berry! By using cooking methods that draw out natural flavors, along with seasonings that increase palatability, you can foster a love of vegetables in the youngest eaters. It's best to serve the zucchini as wedges rather than cubes for safety.

1. Preheat the oven to 425°F.

2. Line a baking sheet with parchment paper or foil. If using foil, spray it generously with olive oil.

3. Combine the Parmesan and garlic powder in a small bowl.

4. In a large bowl, toss the zucchini in the olive oil, then roll the wedges in the seasoning, leaving some to sprinkle on top of the zucchini when it's placed on the baking sheet.

5. Bake until golden brown, 10 to 15 minutes.

6. For crispy pieces, broil for 2 to 3 minutes.

CHANGE IT UP: To introduce more flavors, you may add these ingredients:
- 1 teaspoon of Italian seasoning
- ½ teaspoon of paprika (sweet or smoked)
- ½ teaspoon of rosemary
- Freshly chopped parsley leaves, for garnish

PURÉE TIP: Cook until soft, skipping step 6, then blend with low-sodium broth, formula, or expressed breast milk to desired texture.

BAKED FALAFEL

GLUTEN-FREE OPTION **NUT-FREE** VEGETARIAN VEGAN OPTION

**YIELDS 12
SERVINGS**

1 tablespoon olive oil,
plus more for greasing
and drizzling

1 (15.5-ounce) can
chickpeas, drained
and rinsed

1 small
onion, chopped

1 tablespoon
chopped fresh parsley

2 garlic
cloves, chopped

1 large egg (flax egg
for vegan option)

2 teaspoons
ground cumin

½ teaspoon salt

Pinch black pepper

1 teaspoon
lemon juice

1 teaspoon
baking powder

¾ to 1 cup bread
crumbs (gluten-
free bread crumbs
optional)

Falafel is a savory and nutritious dish from the Middle East. It's often paired with Hummus (page 89), Tzatziki (page 161), or tahini sauce and served in a pita with cucumbers and tomatoes. Garbanzo beans, also called chickpeas, are a wonderful natural source of folate, which is great for brain development and heart health. This recipe was inspired by A Love Letter to Food.

1. Preheat the oven to 400°F. Line a baking sheet with parchment paper or foil. If using foil, coat it generously with olive oil.

2. Combine the chickpeas, onion, parsley, garlic, egg, cumin, salt, pepper, lemon juice, baking powder, and 1 tablespoon of olive oil in a food processor. If you don't have a food processor, you may use a blender to dice the onion, parsley, and garlic, then mash the ingredients together with a potato masher until they form a thick paste.

3. Put the mixture in a large mixing bowl, then add bread crumbs until the mixture is no longer sticky and holds together.

4. Use your hands to form about 1 tablespoon of the mixture into a ball, then slightly flatten it into a patty.

5. Lay the patties on the prepared baking sheet, drizzle with additional olive oil, then bake for 10 minutes on each side.

6. Broil for 1 to 2 minutes on each side.

7. Let cool and enjoy.

TO REFRIGERATE: Store in a sealed container for up to 3 days.

TO FREEZE: Store in an airtight container for up to a month.

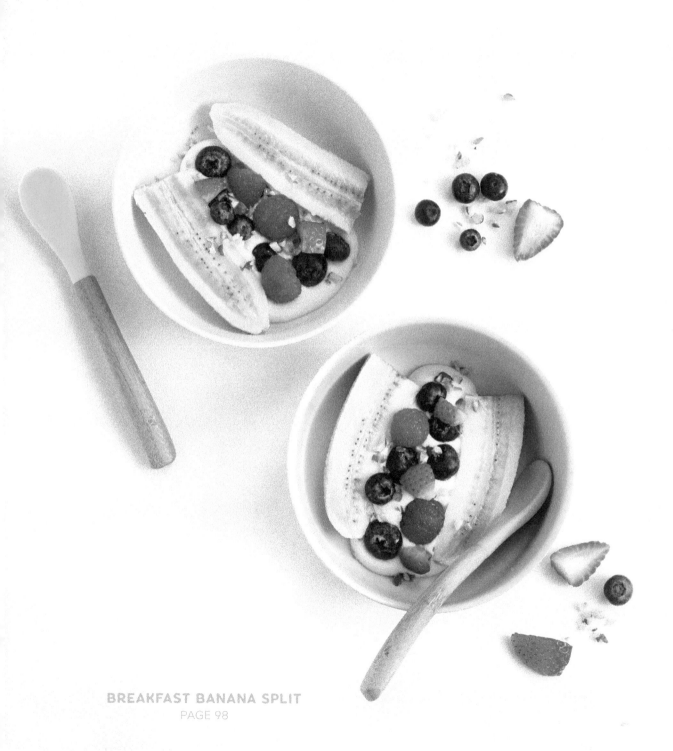

BREAKFAST BANANA SPLIT
PAGE 98

9 TO 12 MONTHS
STAGE THREE GUIDE AND RECIPES

At nine months, your baby is really starting to move. They might be crawling, pulling themselves up to stand, and getting much better at picking up smaller objects, including food, with that pincer grasp. At this point, if you've chosen to use purées, you'll progress to finger foods and other recognizable meals. Your baby will welcome the colors, textures, and overall meal experience as they share in family meals alongside their favorite person—you!

RECIPES 89

SNACKS

BREAKFAST

LUNCH AND DINNER

BABY AT THIS STAGE

Exploration, including food exploration, is key for brain development. What is your curious little one up to now?

DEVELOPMENTAL SKILLS

Until this point, your baby has been using their whole hand to grip toys, foods, and likely your hair. Beginning at nine months, the newly developed pincer grasp allows your baby to pick up smaller items, such as cereal. Your baby is also starting to interact with you more as their language skills develop. They'll start to blow bubbles or to giggle to make you smile.

NUTRITIONAL NEEDS

Breast milk or formula remains the primary source of nutrition for your baby until they are closer to 12 months old. From 9 to 12 months, your baby will drink six to eight ounces, three or four times a day. How much nutrition your child needs will vary from meal to meal and from day to day. If you're concerned about your child's nutrition or growth, speak to your pediatrician or pediatric dietitian.

Iron, zinc, and vitamin D remain important nutrients that are not provided by breast milk. Formula is often fortified with these nutrients, but exposing your little one to a variety of different foods comes with many benefits, so it's still best to offer diverse foods.

WHAT TO INTRODUCE

Right now, your little food explorer finds everything fresh and fascinating. Support that attitude by offering food with a variety of colors, flavors, and textures.

FOODS AND FLAVORS

Everything is exciting and new at this stage. Be sure to introduce your baby to all kinds of foods, including some foods that you don't enjoy—they might have different flavor preferences than you do.

To help your baby progress in developing their pincer grasp, introduce foods like peas, berries that have been cut in half, and small cereals that give lots of practice. It's best to give these alongside foods that are easier to grip so the baby doesn't get frustrated while trying this new skill. Refer to the baby-led feeding recipes in chapters 2 and 3 for ideas.

TOOLS AND UTENSILS

As your baby continues to use age-appropriate utensils, their proficiency will continue to improve. It is still common, and developmentally appropriate, for your baby to use their hands as their utensil skills continue to develop. The tools previously mentioned remain appropriate, but you can also find useful products at discount stores, like Ikea, Amazon, Target, and Walmart. Deciding on a utensil, much like choosing a pacifier or comfort toy, can require some experimentation. See chapter 2 for the main features to look for in a utensil.

You'll continue to use child-size utensils until your baby is around two years old.

TYPICAL MEALS AND SCHEDULE

As your baby grows, their ideal portion size continues to be the size of their fist, a rule that actually continues into adulthood! That's not the total amount that your baby will eat at a meal, but a frame of reference to remember how tiny your baby's tummy is. Your baby might have a single portion at a meal or might eat multiple servings. Let their appetite lead the way.

A meal should include two or three different items, but it doesn't have to be fancy. Some thawed frozen vegetables, a Chocolate Bloomie (page 76), and a piece of cheese provide fiber, fat, protein, and micronutrients, as well as a variety of textures, colors, and flavors. A snack is a miniature meal and should be composed of two different items. Toast with Nut Butter (page 42) is a good example.

Although each family will follow a different schedule, a typical schedule for this stage might look like this (see the Resources on page 191 for a link to alternative schedules). Your baby will be awake for longer stretches at this point.

6:00 A.M.	Wake and feed (breast milk or formula)
7:45 A.M.	Solid food breakfast
8:00 A.M.	Nap (45 to 60 minutes or more)
9:00 A.M.	Wake and feed (breast milk or formula)
9:45 A.M.	Snack option #1
12:00 P.M.	Nap (1½ to 2 hours or more)
2:00 P.M.	Wake and feed (breast milk or formula)
2:45 P.M.	Snack option #2
5:00 P.M.	Solid food dinner
5:30 P.M.	Begin bedtime routine
6:00 P.M.	Breast milk or formula, then to bed

LEARNING TO USE CUPS AND UTENSILS

Sippy cups, straw cups, 360 cups, and more. There are many options out there, but I advise parents to stick with the models that make an easy transition to big-kid versions while following advice from pediatric dentists. A soft-tipped straw cup is easy on a baby's teeth and looks a lot like the cup they'll use as a big kid. Many parents report success with straw cups after going to a coffeehouse and getting a kid-size cup of water for their child to try as they enjoy their own beverage from a very similar cup.

In chapter 1, I suggested giving your baby an open cup for bath-time play. Your child may be proficient enough by this point to try an open cup at the table. If this is new, consider giving them a small cup, perhaps a light plastic shot glass, for practice. This age is a great time to start, because the American Academy of Pediatrics recommends ditching the bottle by 18 months.

Here are some tips and tricks to make this transition go smoothly:

- Let your child pick their own cup; consider bright colors and loved characters.

- Model the new skill by drinking from a similar cup along with your child.

- Make it a game by toasting with your child.

COMMON CHALLENGES

YOUR CHILD ISN'T EATING ENOUGH OR IS EATING TOO MUCH: Your baby was born understanding appetite, but at this point in their development, they may start trying to make you happy—by eating more or less than they might if left to their own biological signals. Create a pressure-free environment at the table. Sit and enjoy a meal with your baby, without encouraging them to eat a specific amount or celebrating each bite.

YOUR CHILD IS THROWING FOOD ON THE GROUND: As your child's language is developing, it's still easier for them to communicate with their hands. When your child throws food, they are indicating they're no longer interested in mealtime. Take them out of their seat and continue with another activity. As you pay close attention, you may notice a look or an action that occurs prior to your baby throwing food, and you can avoid a messy floor by ending the meal at that sign.

YOUR CHILD TAKES A LONG TIME TO EAT AND SEEMS TO CHEW EXCESSIVELY: Start by checking the schedule—allow two to three hours between meals and snacks so your baby can develop an appetite. Offer foods appropriate for your child's development; foods that are difficult to pick up or chew can cause frustration. Although your child may just need more practice, muscle weakness in the tongue, jaw, or cheeks can cause difficulty chewing or swallowing, resulting in excessive chewing and lengthy, frustrating meals. Speak to your pediatrician if you're concerned. Additionally, here are some tips for reducing the chances of overstimulation at the table:

* Avoid books, TV, and toys at the table.

* Present a calm and positive atmosphere.

* Provide appropriate portion sizes.

HUMMUS THREE WAYS

GLUTEN-FREE **NUT-FREE** **VEGAN**

YIELDS 6 (⅓-CUP)
SERVINGS

1 (15.5-ounce) can
chickpeas, drained
and rinsed

⅓ cup tahini

2 tablespoons
lemon juice

2 or 3 garlic cloves

2 tablespoons olive oil

Pinch cumin

Pinch kosher salt

2 tablespoons seltzer

The hummus trend has really taken off in recent years. It's no surprise when you learn how great tahini and chickpeas are for growing brains and how versatile a basic hummus recipe can be. Hummus works as a spread on toast, as a dip, or as finger paint for a hesitant eater (no, that's not a joke—it's a method of introduction). Start with a basic hummus recipe, and keep reading for a couple of flavor twists.

CLASSIC HUMMUS

1. Blend the chickpeas, tahini, lemon juice, garlic, olive oil, cumin, and salt in a food processor or blender. You may need to turn off the machine and scrape down the sides once or twice.

2. Blend to desired consistency, adding the seltzer to help thin as needed. If you don't have seltzer, water or the liquid from the can of chickpeas works well.

CONTINUED

SPINACH PESTO HUMMUS

4 cups spinach, fresh or frozen

¼ cup fresh basil or 2 to 3 teaspoons frozen basil, diced

Make Classic Hummus (page 89), blending in spinach and basil.

ROASTED RED PEPPER HUMMUS

6 ounces jarred roasted red bell peppers (or 1 to 2 roasted red bell peppers)

Make Classic Hummus (page 89), blending in roasted red bell peppers.

TO REFRIGERATE: Store in a tightly sealed container for up to 4 days.

TO FREEZE: Store in a freezer-safe, airtight container, leaving some space at the top. Cover with a layer of plastic wrap, seal, and cover with plastic wrap again. Freeze for up to 4 months.

SAFETY TIP: If you or your baby has a tahini allergy, you may replace the tahini with peanut butter, cashew butter, or sunflower seed butter.

COOKING TIP: Dried basil will not work well in the Spinach Pesto Hummus.

YOGURT-COVERED BLUEBERRY KABOBS

GLUTEN-FREE **NUT-FREE** VEGETARIAN VEGAN OPTION

YIELDS 3 SKEWERS

1 pint fresh blueberries

1 cup plain full-fat Greek yogurt (yogurt alternative for vegan option)

TO FREEZE: Follow instructions up to step 4. Then put frozen skewers into a freezer-safe container or freezer bag. Keep for up to 3 months.

Blueberries and yogurt are both delicious. Why not combine them and increase their fun factor by serving them on a stick? You can use a standard bamboo skewer, using a strong pair of scissors to cut off the sharp point, or a wooden coffee stirrer. If you use a larger berry, such as a strawberry, opt for an ice pop stick. This is a fun snack to enjoy with your child, allowing you to demonstrate safety skills while you both enjoy a tasty treat. Consider including your child in the fun of skewering the blueberries—but be prepared with some extra blueberries as some (or most) won't make it onto the stick.

1. Prepare a baking sheet by lining it with parchment paper, foil, or wax paper.

2. Wash the blueberries carefully, showing your child how the berries "take a bath," then pat dry.

3. Thread some blueberries onto your chosen stick, then roll in yogurt.

4. Lay the skewers in a single layer on the prepared baking sheet, then freeze for at least an hour, until the yogurt has hardened.

5. Let thaw for about 5 minutes before enjoying.

CHANGE IT UP:
- Try substituting strawberries, raspberries, or blackberries.
- Prior to freezing, sprinkle the berries with finely chopped nuts or seeds.

APPLE COOKIES

GLUTEN-FREE **NUT-FREE OPTION** **VEGAN**

YIELDS 5 COOKIES

1 apple (skin on or off)

3 tablespoons peanut butter or other nut or seed butter, room temperature

2 tablespoons topping (hemp seeds, sunflower seeds, finely chopped nuts, toasted shredded coconut)

Eating sliced apples has never been so much fun. This is another recipe where you can involve the kids. Try spreading the nut or seed butter using a hand-over-hand method. Allow your child to select toppings and sprinkle them on top of the apple. By slicing the apple thinly, you avoid the large chunks of raw apple that can be a choking hazard at this age.

1. Slice the apple thinly to make about 5 apple rounds.

2. Spread the nut or seed butter over each apple slice.

3. Sprinkle the toppings on top of the apple slices.

TO REFRIGERATE: If you plan to make these for later, spray the apple slices with diluted lemon juice (half lemon juice and half water) to help the apples keep their color, then decorate your "cookies" and cover. Refrigerate for no more than a day.

BAKED TOFU WITH DIPPING SAUCE

GLUTEN-FREE OPTION **NUT-FREE** VEGAN

YIELDS 6 TO 8 SERVINGS

1 tablespoon olive oil

3 tablespoons maple syrup

1 tablespoon sesame oil

2 tablespoons soy sauce (tamari for gluten-free option)

2 garlic cloves, diced

¼ teaspoon ground ginger or ½ teaspoon grated fresh ginger

1 block firm tofu, pressed and cubed

Tofu is a great source of protein and calcium. Tofu tends to take on the flavor of the marinade, so be sure to pick something very tasty. Although tofu gets a bad rap along with many other soy-based foods, there is actually no risk of hormonal disruption—tofu, soy milk, soy sauce, and soy beans are safe and nutritious. For more information on soy, see Nap Time Nutrition in the Resources (page 189) Serve this recipe over rice or in veggie-filled lettuce wraps.

1. Preheat the oven to 425°F.

2. Prepare a baking sheet by lining it with foil and lightly coating it with the olive oil.

3. In a small bowl, mix the maple syrup, sesame oil, soy sauce, garlic, and ginger together. Marinate the tofu in half of the sauce and reserve the rest for dipping.

4. Lay out the tofu on the prepared baking sheet and bake for 10 minutes on each side. Let it cool before serving.

TO REFRIGERATE: Store in a sealed container for up to 4 days.

CHANGE IT UP: Serve tofu in a lettuce wrap by adding shredded carrots, mung bean sprouts, chopped mango, and shredded purple cabbage.

SEASONAL SMOOTHIES

GLUTEN-FREE **NUT-FREE OPTION** **VEGETARIAN** **VEGAN OPTION**

YIELDS 2 TO 3 SERVINGS

Smoothies are a great choice, no matter the season. By starting with a standard base formula, you can change up the flavors and the nutrition while remaining confident that the final product will be delicious. During the hot summer months, consider using an ice pop tray and freezing your smoothies into a tasty afternoon treat. To prep your smoothie the night before, add the solid ingredients to a freezer bag and store in the freezer. Then, dump the contents of the bag into the blender, add the liquid, and blend. Protein powders are not usually recommended for children, but see the tips for optional nutrition boosts.

SMOOTHIE BASE

1 banana

1½ cups fruit of your choice

½ to 1 cup vegetables

½ cup liquid

½ cup ice

CHOCOLATE AND PEANUT BUTTER SMOOTHIE

1 banana

1 tablespoon creamy peanut butter or seed butter

¼ cup milk (milk alternative for vegan option)

¼ cup plain full-fat Greek yogurt (yogurt alternative for vegan option)

1 tablespoon cocoa powder

½ cup ice

VERY BERRY BLAST

1 banana

1½ cups blueberries, raspberries, and strawberries

1 cup spinach

½ cup orange juice or pineapple juice

½ cup ice

MORNING SUNRISE

1 banana

¼ cup butternut squash purée

1 mango, peeled, pitted, and cut into chunks

½ cup orange juice

½ cup ice

GREEN GOODNESS

1 banana

1 cup spinach

1 whole orange, peeled and pulled into segments

½ cup pineapple juice

½ cup ice

Put all the ingredients for the smoothie in a blender and blend to desired consistency.

TO REFRIGERATE: Store in a sealed cup. Stir before serving.

NUTRITION TIP: Consider adding ¼ avocado to increase the fat content or ¼ block of soft tofu to increase calcium and protein.

BAKED OATMEAL CUPS

GLUTEN-FREE **NUT-FREE** VEGETARIAN VEGAN OPTION

**YIELDS 12
MUFFIN CUPS**

Nonstick cooking
spray (optional)

2 ripe
bananas, mashed

½ cup applesauce

¼ cup maple syrup

2 large eggs (flax eggs
for vegan option)

1 teaspoon
vanilla extract

3 cups old-
fashioned oats

2 teaspoons
cinnamon

1 teaspoon
baking powder

½ teaspoon salt

TO FREEZE: Store in
an airtight container
for up to 4 months.

Oatmeal cups make a wonderful breakfast or snack on the go. They can easily be prepped and stored in the fridge or the freezer, and they can be served warm or cold. This recipe also contains some galactogogues, which help support milk supply in a nursing mother.

1. Preheat the oven to 350°F. Spray a muffin tin with nonstick cooking spray or line with paper liners.

2. In a large bowl, mix the mashed banana, applesauce, maple syrup, eggs, and vanilla.

3. In another bowl, mix the oats, cinnamon, baking powder, and salt.

4. Add the dry ingredients to the wet ingredients and mix until just combined.

5. Use a ¼-cup measuring cup to fill the muffin cups to about three-quarters full.

6. Bake for 20 to 25 minutes. Allow to cool before serving.

TO REFRIGERATE: Store in an airtight container for up to 4 days.

CHANGE IT UP: Create a new experience by adding ⅓ cup of dried blueberries, chopped dried apples, or chocolate chips.

FRUIT AND YOGURT PARFAIT

GLUTEN-FREE OPTION **NUT-FREE OPTION** VEGETARIAN VEGAN OPTION

YIELDS 2 SERVINGS

1 cup plain full-fat Greek yogurt (yogurt alternative for vegan option)

1 cup mixed berries, fresh or frozen

Additional toppings: granola, crushed nuts, shredded coconut, sliced banana, Coconut Whipped Cream (page 98)

CHANGE IT UP: Try going tropical with mango, papaya, and kiwifruit.

Parfait is a French word meaning "perfect." A parfait is perfect because it meets your needs exactly—some contain granola and nuts, and some are simply fruit and yogurt. Let family members build their own perfect parfaits by serving this dish deconstructed. When your child is still too young to handle serving themselves, they can indicate what they would like with a smile, giggle, or even an interested look. This recipe can be a messy endeavor, so it may be best to serve just before bath time. For extra fun, serve the parfaits in an ice cream cone!

1. Layer the ingredients in cups or bowls. Consider using transparent dishes so everyone can enjoy seeing the layers.

2. Top with desired toppings.

TO REFRIGERATE: Store in a sealed container for 2 to 3 days. Refrigerate ingredients separately.

NUTRITION TIP: Round out the meal even more by adding ½ cup of quinoa.

SAFETY TIP: Any round fruit, such as cherries or grapes, should be cut in half lengthwise.

COTTAGE CHEESE MUFFINS

GLUTEN-FREE OPTION **NUT-FREE** VEGETARIAN

**YIELDS 12 TO
15 MUFFINS**

Nonstick cooking
spray (optional)

2 cups small curd full-
fat cottage cheese

8 tablespoons
(1 stick) unsalted
butter, melted

3 large eggs, beaten

6 tablespoons white
or brown sugar

Pinch of salt (unless
cottage cheese has
added salt)

1 teaspoon pumpkin
pie spice

Pinch nutmeg or
allspice

1½ cups all-purpose
flour (gluten-free flour
optional)

2 teaspoons
baking powder

TO REFRIGERATE:
Store in a sealed con-
tainer for 3 to 5 days.

Inspired by Daniella Silver's *The Silver Platter*, this one-bowl muffin recipe can be made fruity by adding blueberries or peaches, or it can be made savory by reducing the sugar and adding sun-dried tomatoes. This muffin is more like a hearty soufflé. Although the muffins can easily be stored in the fridge or freezer, eating them fresh out of the oven is an experience you won't want to miss.

1. Preheat the oven to 350°F.

2. Line a muffin pan with paper liners or spray with the cooking spray, if using.

3. In a large mixing bowl, stir the cottage cheese, butter, eggs, sugar, salt, pumpkin pie spice, nutmeg, and flour until well combined.

4. Sprinkle the baking powder over the dough and mix until incorporated.

5. Using a ¼-cup measuring cup, scoop the batter into the prepared muffin tins.

6. Bake for 35 minutes, until the tops are golden brown.

TO FREEZE: Store in an airtight, freezer-safe container for up to 2 months.

CHANGE IT UP: Make this dish your own with one of these flavor-shifting options:

• Add in 1 cup of blueberries, peaches, or strawberries.

• Reduce the sugar to 3 tablespoons and add ¼ cup of chopped sun-dried tomatoes.

• Sprinkle some Cheddar cheese on top of the muffins before baking.

BREAKFAST BANANA SPLIT

GLUTEN-FREE **NUT-FREE OPTION** **VEGAN**

YIELDS 2 SERVINGS

1 (14-ounce) can
full-fat coconut milk,
refrigerated upside
down overnight

1 teaspoon
vanilla extract

1 banana

½ cup mixed berries,
fresh or frozen

¼ cup toppings
(shelled hemp seeds,
sunflower seeds,
finely chopped nuts,
shredded coconut)

Take a banana split to the breakfast table with this filling and nutritious meal. You can serve it to look like a traditional banana split, or you can serve it parfait-style. The coconut whips up best if you chill the mixing bowl and whisk or beaters in the freezer or in an ice bath for 30 minutes before using. You'll need electric beaters or an electric whisk for this recipe.

1. Scoop out ¾ cup of the solid cream from the refrigerated coconut milk can. Reserve the rest of the liquid for another recipe, like the Seasonal Smoothies (page 94).

2. Put the coconut cream in a chilled medium-size mixing bowl. Whisk or beat the coconut cream for about a minute. It should look like whipped cream. Sometimes the cream looks curdled and grainy before whipping up—just keep whipping.

3. Fold in the vanilla extract and continue to beat on low speed until incorporated.

4. Peel the banana and slice lengthwise or into rounds. Place the sliced banana in a dish, add the coconut whipped cream, then add the berries and desired toppings.

TO REFRIGERATE: Store in a sealed container for up to 3 days.

CHIA PUDDING PARFAIT

GLUTEN-FREE **NUT-FREE** VEGAN

YIELDS 2 SERVINGS

1 (14-ounce) can full-fat coconut milk, room temperature

⅓ cup chia seeds

1 tablespoon maple syrup

½ cup berries

1 large banana, sliced

CHANGE IT UP:
For chocolate chia pudding, add a pinch of salt and 3 table-spoons of cocoa powder before setting overnight.

Chia was first made famous in the United States during the 1980s, when people spread it on ceramic animals and grew it as a house plant. It has since made a resurgence in edible form. Chia seeds are high in both soluble and insoluble fiber. They can replace eggs in some baked recipes, and they add a crunch to granola. In this recipe, the chia seeds give the parfait a texture that's similar to tapioca pudding. This recipe makes extra pudding to save for later, too.

1. In a small mixing bowl, stir together the coconut milk, chia seeds, and maple syrup.

2. After five minutes, stir the ingredients again.

3. Let the mixture set overnight.

4. Serve with the berries and sliced banana.

TO REFRIGERATE: Store in an airtight container for up to 3 days.

COOKING TIP: For a smoother texture, blend the set chia pudding in a strong blender.

CHEESY BAKED EGGS

GLUTEN-FREE **NUT-FREE** **VEGETARIAN**

YIELDS 6 EGGS

6 large eggs

3 slices cheese
or 6 teaspoons
Parmesan cheese

TO REFRIGERATE:
Store in a sealed container for up to 2 days.

This is possibly the easiest egg recipe you'll find. You can even make these eggs before you've had your coffee. They can be made ahead of time and reheated in the microwave, or they can be eaten fresh. It's amazing how baking brings out the egg's subtle savory quality that you didn't even know you were missing.

1. Preheat the oven to 375°F. Line a muffin pan with paper or silicone liners.

2. Crack an egg into each muffin cup.

3. Place ½ slice of cheese or 1 teaspoon of Parmesan cheese on top of each egg.

4. Bake for 20 to 22 minutes, until the eggs are set.

5. Remove from the oven, let them cool, and enjoy!

TO FREEZE: Let the eggs cool completely, then put them in a freezer bag, remove all the air, and freeze for up to 3 months.

CHANGE IT UP:
- Scramble the eggs before baking.
- Add some veggies. Use a spiralizer or peeler to make ribbons out of zucchini or sweet potato. Put 2 ribbons in the bottom of the liner, then add the egg and cheese. Bake as directed.

HOMEMADE CHICKEN FINGERS

GLUTEN-FREE OPTION **NUT-FREE**

YIELDS 8 SERVINGS

Olive oil cooking spray (optional)

1½ cups panko bread crumbs (gluten-free bread crumbs optional)

½ teaspoon onion powder

Pinch of salt

1 large egg

1 pound boneless, skinless chicken breast or thighs, cut into ½-inch-thick slices

1 tablespoon olive oil

Homemade chicken fingers are much easier to make than you might think. For added nutrition, dip them in Veggieful Sauce (page 73) or in any of the hummus options (page 89). And ketchup is always a big hit with kids. Make a big batch of these chicken fingers and freeze them for another easy meal. For added fun, cuddle on the couch with your kids and watch the YouTube clip on how panko bread crumbs are made!

1. Preheat the oven to 400°F.

2. Prepare a baking sheet by lining it with parchment paper or foil. If using foil, spray it with the cooking spray.

3. In a medium-size mixing bowl, combine the bread crumbs, onion powder, and salt. Then spread this mixture onto a plate or another baking sheet.

4. In another medium-size mixing bowl, beat the egg.

5. Place the chicken pieces in the bowl with the egg and toss to coat each piece.

CONTINUED

6. Add each piece of chicken to the plate with the bread crumbs, then roll each piece to cover in the crumbs and seasoning.

7. Place the breaded chicken on the prepared baking sheet and coat with the olive oil.

8. Bake for 25 minutes, flipping halfway through. The internal temperature of the chicken should reach 165°F.

TO REFRIGERATE: Store in a sealed container for 3 to 4 days.

TO FREEZE: Store in an airtight container for up to 3 months.

CHANGE IT UP: Try adding ¼ teaspoon of garlic powder, ¼ teaspoon of thyme, and ¼ teaspoon of parsley or ¼ teaspoon of paprika to your bread crumbs.

SAFETY TIP: Serve the chicken in strips, not in very small pieces. A very small piece can be a choking hazard, and serving the chicken in strips will help your child learn to take the right size bite.

BLACK BEAN BURGERS

GLUTEN-FREE OPTION **NUT-FREE** VEGETARIAN VEGAN OPTION

YIELDS 8
SMALL BURGERS

Olive oil cooking spray (optional)

1 (15-ounce) can black beans, drained and rinsed

½ bell pepper, finely chopped

½ small onion, finely chopped

2 garlic cloves, peeled and chopped, or 2 teaspoons diced garlic

1 teaspoon cumin

Pinch salt

Pinch pepper

1 large egg (flax egg for vegan option)

⅔ to 1 cup whole-wheat or panko bread crumbs (gluten-free bread crumbs optional)

Veggie burgers are a great way to round out a meal. You can make a couple of batches and freeze them for a quick dinner for those days when you get caught in traffic or you just don't feel like cooking. You can double the size and serve them on a bun like a classic burger or make them smaller to accompany a salad.

1. Preheat the oven to 375°F.

2. Prepare a baking sheet by lining it with parchment paper or foil. If using foil, spray it with the cooking spray.

3. Place the beans in a large mixing bowl and mash with a potato masher until just chunky.

4. Add the bell pepper, onion, garlic, cumin, salt, and pepper to the bowl.

5. Add the egg and ⅔ cup of bread crumbs to the mixture. Mix well. If the mixture seems too wet, add more bread crumbs as needed.

6. Form 8 balls and press lightly into patties.

7. Bake on the prepared baking sheet for 7 to 8 minutes, flip, then bake for another 7 minutes.

TO REFRIGERATE: Store in a sealed container for up to 3 days.

TO FREEZE: Place in an airtight container. Layer parchment paper between layers of burgers, wrap with foil, and store for up to 3 months.

MOROCCAN ROASTED CHICKPEAS

GLUTEN-FREE **NUT-FREE** **VEGAN**

**YIELDS 12
SERVINGS**

¼ cup olive oil

5 large
tomatoes, chopped

5 garlic cloves,
minced, or
5 teaspoons jarred
minced garlic

1 tablespoon paprika

Pinch salt

Pinch pepper

2 (15.5-ounce) cans
chickpeas, drained
and rinsed

1 red bell
pepper, chopped

PURÉE TIP: At
step 4, bake covered
for 1 hour, let cool,
and purée.

Chickpeas are a staple in my house. Whether I'm making these savory roasted chickpeas, Hummus (page 89), or Chickpea Blondies (page 162), on any given day, I'm probably cooking with beans. This dish is wonderful as a side to salmon or chicken, or with a salad for a light meal. It also pairs well with rice, and you can serve it warm or cold. You can make this recipe in one pan if you use a large cast iron pan.

1. Preheat the oven to 350°F.

2. In a cast iron skillet, heat the oil and sauté the tomatoes, garlic, paprika, salt, and pepper for about 10 minutes.

3. Mix in the chickpeas and bell pepper.

4. Bake in the cast iron skillet in the oven for about 1½ hours, until most of the liquid has evaporated. If using a nonstick skillet, transfer beans to a baking sheet lined with parchment paper before baking.

TO REFRIGERATE: Store in a sealed container for up to 5 days.

CHANGE IT UP: If you're making this for kids who appreciate some heat, you can replace the bell pepper with 1 to 2 jalapeños.

SWEETS AND BEETS

GLUTEN-FREE **NUT-FREE** VEGAN

**YIELDS 4 TO 6
SERVINGS**

Nonstick cooking
spray (optional)

1 medium beet,
peeled and cut into
½-inch cubes

1 large sweet potato,
peeled and cut into
½-inch cubes

1 tablespoon olive oil

½ teaspoon
garlic powder

½ teaspoon salt

PURÉE TIP: Reduce
the salt to ¼ tea-
spoon. After step 3,
let the cubes cool
and purée.

Beets are a common food in Eastern Europe but are often overlooked in North America. Their earthy, sweet flavor pairs nicely with sweet pota-toes and will be a hit with kids of all ages. Avoid beet-stained hands by using gloves.

1. Preheat the oven to 400°F. Line a baking sheet with parchment paper or spray it with the nonstick cooking spray.

2. Arrange the beet and sweet potato cubes on the baking sheet and toss wih the oil, garlic powder, and salt.

3. Roast for 20 minutes, flip, and roast for another 20 minutes.

4. Serve warm or at room temperature.

TO REFRIGERATE: Store in a sealed container for up to 3 days.

TO FREEZE: Store in an airtight container, such as a zip-top freezer bag, for up to 3 months.

PEANUT BUTTER AND BANANA SUSHI

GLUTEN-FREE OPTION **NUT-FREE OPTION** VEGAN

YIELDS 3 SERVINGS

2 tablespoons peanut butter or other nut or seed butter

1 (12-inch) tortilla (gluten-free tortilla optional)

1 banana

SAFETY TIP: Large chunks of nut and seed butter can be a choking hazard, so be sure to spread nut or seed butter evenly across the tortilla before rolling.

TO REFRIGERATE: Store in an airtight container for 1 day.

This quick and easy recipe can be adapted as your child grows. Banana is a popular food among new eaters, and this recipe rounds out the meal by safely including some nut or seed butter. For best results, buy a tortilla that bends easily without cracking—warming up your tortillas for a few seconds in the microwave may help them bend. If you accidentally buy one that cracks, make the sushi quesadilla-style!

1. Spread the peanut butter in a thin layer over the whole tortilla surface.

2. Lay the banana on one end and roll up the tortilla.

3. Slice the "sushi" roll into 1-inch pieces and serve.

CHANGE IT UP:

• Any nut or seed butter will work with this recipe.

• Make lollipops out of the slices by pushing an ice pop stick through the side.

• You can use a piece of sandwich bread, rolled out thinly—have your child participate in the rolling!

• Try adding toasted coconut, mini dark chocolate chips, chia seeds, sunflower seeds, or chopped dried fruit.

SANDWICH KABOBS

GLUTEN-FREE OPTION **NUT-FREE OPTION** VEGETARIAN OPTION VEGAN OPTION

YIELDS 3 KABOBS

1 sandwich

1 handful fruit/ veggie/cheese accompaniment

TO REFRIGERATE: Store in a sealed container for 1 to 2 days.

A sandwich is a sandwich, but a sandwich kabob is a party! You can make this concept work with almost any sandwich, pairing the fruits or veggies to match the sandwich flavor profile. These kabobs fit nicely into lunch boxes when you use a coffee stirrer for the stick.

- PB&J with strawberries
- Turkey and cheese with cherry tomatoes, halved lengthwise
- Cream cheese and cucumber with grapes, halved lengthwise
- Peanut Butter and Banana Sushi (page 106) with raspberries
- Grilled cheese with bell pepper spears

1. Using a pizza slicer or a sharp knife, cut your sandwich into 9 bite-size pieces.

2. Skewer each sandwich piece on a wooden coffee stirrer with the fruit, veggie, or cheese accompaniment between pieces.

SAFETY TIPS:

- Be sure that anything round, such as cherry tomatoes or grapes, is cut in half lengthwise to prevent a choking hazard.
- Use a wooden coffee stirrer or a bamboo kabob skewer with the pointed tip cut off.

VEGGIE DUMPLINGS

NUT-FREE VEGAN

**YIELDS 32
DUMPLINGS**

1 tablespoon olive oil

1 garlic clove,
chopped, or
1 teaspoon of jarred
minced garlic

4 cups shredded
cabbage and carrot

10 green
onions, chopped

1 teaspoon sesame oil

2 tablespoons low-
sodium soy sauce

1 package wonton
wraps (with at least
32 wrappers)

TO REFRIGERATE:
Store in an airtight
container, ideally
not touching, for up
to 2 days.

TO FREEZE: Lay in
a single layer on a
baking tray and freeze
for about an hour.
Then transfer the
dumplings to a freezer
bag and store for up
to 2 months.

Dumplings are often overlooked as a make-at-home option, but they are so easy to make, and they fit so nicely in a little kid's tiny fist. This recipe is also a fun opportunity to start working on those chopstick skills by getting child-size, child-friendly chopsticks—although your expectations should be low. Using novel utensils is a fun and creative way to keep mealtimes entertaining and engaging. Wonton wraps are great to keep on hand. You can store them in the freezer and bust them out when the mood hits. This is a forgiving recipe, so don't worry if you're a bit short on any one ingredient.

1. Using a large nonstick pan or wok, heat the oil over medium heat, then sauté the garlic and the cabbage-and-carrot blend until the cabbage begins to shrink, 2 to 3 minutes.

2. Add the green onions, sesame oil, and soy sauce. Continue to cook for about 5 minutes, until the liquid begins to evaporate.

3. Remove the pan from the stovetop and set aside.

4. Fill each wonton wrap with some of the mixture. Follow the dumpling folding instructions on the package. It may take a few tries to get it right.

5. Boil a large pot of water. When the water comes to a rolling boil, cook the dumplings, about 8 at a time, until they are cooked through, 3 to 4 minutes.

6. Use a slotted spoon to remove the dumplings and set on a plate, but don't let them touch. Let cool and enjoy.

CHANGE IT UP: Consider adding 1 tablespoon of finely grated ginger in step 1 or add 2 cups of shiitake mushrooms, chopped, in step 2.

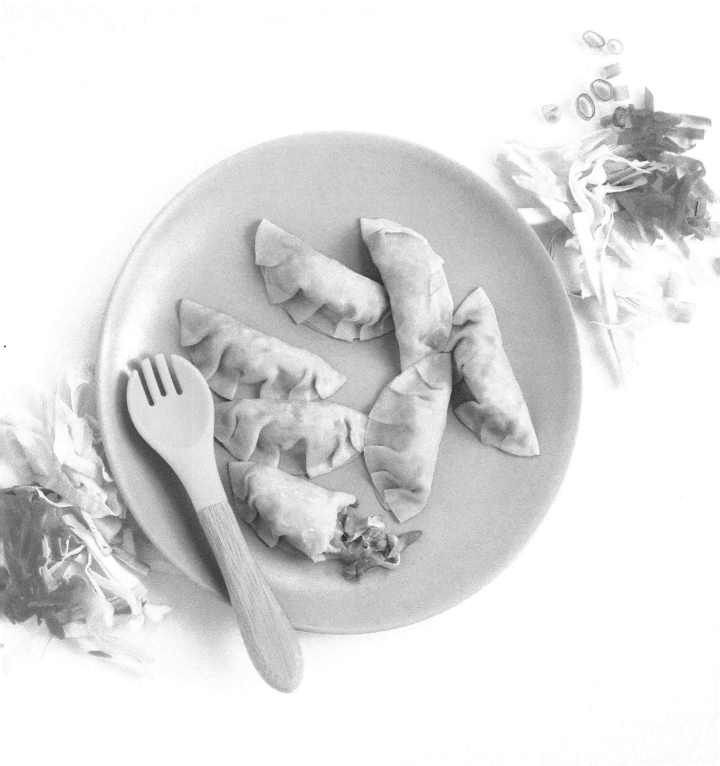

PASTA SALAD

GLUTEN-FREE OPTION **NUT-FREE** **VEGETARIAN** **VEGAN OPTION**

YIELDS 2 SERVINGS

2 ounces pasta, like rotini or fusilli (gluten-free pasta optional)

1 tablespoon olive oil

Small handful of cherry tomatoes, halved or quartered

1 teaspoon Parmesan cheese (nutritional yeast for vegan option)

Pinch dried oregano

Pinch garlic powder

NUTRITION TIP: Consider adding spinach to the mix. Shred the spinach and add to the drained and rinsed pasta while still hot. It will wilt as the pasta cools.

Pasta is such a fun food for kids, since it comes in so many shapes, sizes, and colors. Experiment with different kinds to keep it fun and interesting. Fortified pasta can be a great source of fiber, iron, folate, and other micronutrients. You can choose to provide a fork for exposure and experience, but don't be surprised when your little one's hands dive in.

1. Cook pasta according to the package instructions, drain, and rinse.

2. Toss the pasta in the olive oil and let cool.

3. Mixed the cooled pasta with the tomatoes, cheese, oregano, and garlic powder. Serve and enjoy.

TO REFRIGERATE: Store in a sealed container for up to 3 days.

SAFETY TIP: Cherry and grape tomatoes, olives, or anything of a similar shape should be halved lengthwise before serving.

LEFTOVER MASHED POTATO SOUP

GLUTEN-FREE **NUT-FREE** **VEGAN OPTION**

YIELDS 10 SERVINGS

1 tablespoon olive oil

½ onion, chopped

1 cup leftover mashed potatoes

4 cups low-sodium chicken or vegetable broth

1 zucchini, chopped

1 bell pepper, chopped

1½ cups frozen vegetable mix (carrots, corn, green beans)

It's always great to cut down on food waste, but certain foods, like mashed potatoes, just aren't the same the second time around. By creating something new, like this soup featuring leftover mashed potatoes, limited ingredients can be stretched and enjoyed again by the whole family. White potatoes are high in potassium, vitamin C, vitamin B6, fiber, and more! A trick to cooling soup without diluting it is to add frozen peas, straight out of the bag, to your child's bowl.

1. Heat the oil in a large soup pot over medium heat. Sauté the onion in the oil for 2 to 3 minutes, or until translucent.

2. In a blender, blend the onion, potatoes, and broth.

3. In a pot, rice cooker, slow cooker, or pressure cooker, combine the onion mixture with the zucchini and pepper and heat.

4. Add the frozen mixed veggies to cool the soup and enjoy!

TO FREEZE: Store in an airtight container for up to 6 months.

TO REFRIGERATE: Store in a sealed container for no more than 3 days.

SAFETY TIP: Food should be served warm or at room temperature but not hot. You can test the temperature of the food on the inside of your forearm.

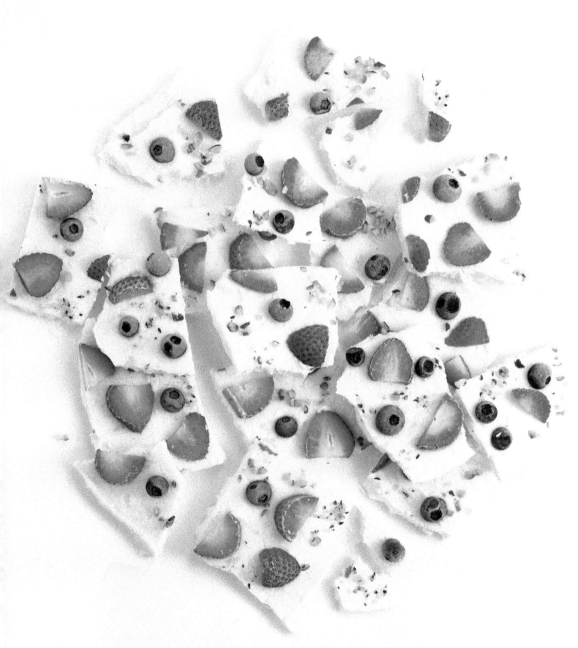

FROZEN YOGURT BARK
PAGE 125

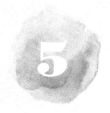

12 TO 18 MONTHS

EARLY TODDLER GUIDE AND RECIPES

Every stage comes with its own brand of fun. Now your toddler is working toward building a vocabulary. Your toddler understands more of what you're saying, and reading together is becoming more fun. Your child may be using more imagination by enjoying some pretend play, such as pretending to cook with little pots and pans, pretending to clean with a little broom, or pretending to drive.

RECIPES 119

SNACKS

BREAKFAST

LUNCH AND DINNER

BABY AT THIS STAGE

As your baby becomes a toddler, their sense of adventure is growing. Big changes are coming.

DEVELOPMENTAL SKILLS

By now your toddler is trying to imitate your use of utensils, which makes it even more important to sit together and enjoy each other's company for meals and snacks. Bring your curious little one into the kitchen for some food prep fun. Consider making Seasonal Smoothies (page 94)—let your child add ingredients to the blender, put the top on, and hit the on button!

NUTRITIONAL NEEDS

When your child reaches 12 months, you can transition them off breast milk and onto full-fat (whole) cow's milk, or a milk alternative. You may also continue pumping or feeding at the breast. The World Health Organization promotes breastfeeding up to two years and beyond, and the American Academy of Pediatrics supports ongoing breastfeeding for as long as it continues to work for both mother and child.

Formula, including toddler-specific formula, is no longer necessary, as it can be replaced by whole milk or a milk substitute. See page 117 for more information on transitioning to cow's milk or milk alternatives.

Until this point, you have provided milk first and food second. When your baby reaches 12 months, you'll prioritize solid food over milk. Provide a cup of milk with meals, and water between meals for hydration. Providing a variety of foods will help you meet your child's nutritional needs. By sticking to your schedule, offering food every two to three hours, and following your toddler's appetite cues, you will meet their nutritional needs.

By following your child's progress on the World Health Organization's growth chart, you'll get a better picture of their overall nutrition and development. If your child was born in the 90th percentile on the growth chart and continues along that trend, you know that their nutrition and growth are appropriate. Likewise, if your child was born in the 5th percentile and continues along that line, you'll know that their nutrition and growth are also appropriate.

WHAT TO INTRODUCE

Variety is key for good nutrition. When your baby reaches the 12-month mark, there are a couple of ingredients that are now appropriate.

FOODS AND FLAVORS

When your baby was under 12 months old, you avoided honey and excess salt. Now honey is permitted, and your toddler can handle more salt.

Now that your child's nutrition depends on solid foods, it's even more important to offer a variety. By including different colors, textures, and flavors, you'll provide a range of macronutrients (carbohydrates, protein, and fat) and micronutrients (vitamins and minerals). Balance isn't possible at every meal but is met over time—over the course of the day or even a couple of days. Meal planning helps you see where to shift foods for better balance.

As your child starts to use their utensils more regularly and independently, you can experiment with what is working and ditch what isn't serving you (pun intended). Since your toddler is paying attention and following your lead, opt for utensils that resemble your own. You can find an array of miniature stainless-steel utensils online. But it's also appropriate to continue to provide the colorful plastic utensils if your child prefers them.

TYPICAL MEALS AND SCHEDULE

The appropriate portion size for your child continues to be the size of their fist. A snack is roughly two servings, and a meal is about three servings, but that doesn't determine how much your child will actually consume. Just like adults, babies, toddlers, and kids have days when they eat more and days when they eat less. Let your child's appetite lead the way.

A typical breakfast might look like a Morning Glory Muffin (page 120), half of a mandarin orange, and a piece of cheese. A snack might be a piece of Frozen Yogurt Bark (page 125) and a few pretzels.

6:00 A.M.	Wake up
6:30 A.M.	Breakfast, including two ounces of whole milk
8:00 A.M.	Nap (45 to 60 minutes or more)
9:15 A.M.	Snack, including two ounces of whole milk
11:30 A.M.	Lunch, including two ounces of whole milk
12:00 P.M.	Nap (1½ to 2 hours or more)
2:30 P.M.	Snack, including two ounces of whole milk
5:00 P.M.	Dinner, including two ounces of whole milk
6:00 P.M.	Bedtime

Although every family has a different dynamic, and therefore a different schedule, when your baby is 12 months old, your schedule might resemble this one. Time awake between naps will be two, three, and four hours as the day progresses.

TRANSITIONING TO COW'S MILK OR A MILK ALTERNATIVE

Some children can transition from breast milk or formula directly to cow's milk without any problems. Others may experience constipation or a general sore tummy. You may slowly introduce cow's milk by first mixing expressed breast milk or formula with ¼ cup of cow's milk and then increasing the amount of cow's milk to ¾ cup over the course of a few days to a week.

Provide about two ounces of whole milk (or milk alternative) at each meal and snack. From 12 to 18 months of age, your toddler will drink 8 to 12 ounces of milk per day. Between meals and snacks, water can provide hydration without impacting your child's appetite for the next meal or snack.

Cow's milk provides important nutrition for your child: calcium, fat, protein, and vitamin D. If your family is dairy-free, there are many alternatives. Soy milk is the preferred alternative since it naturally provides some protein and fat. Almond milk, rice milk, oat milk, pea milk, and hemp milk are other common options. Select a calcium-fortified milk alternative to help with growing bones. Although calcium is in nuts, leafy greens, and fish, the level isn't close to that found in milk or fortified alternative milks.

If you're avoiding dairy, include calcium, vitamin D, and fat in other areas of the diet. The American Academy of Pediatrics recommends vitamin D supplementation of 400 IU daily for babies up to 12 months and 600 IU daily for children and adolescents.

COMMON CHALLENGES

YOUR CHILD PREFERS MILK TO SOLID FOOD: Although milk is healthy, too much milk can result in constipation, iron-deficiency anemia (as too much calcium inhibits iron absorption), and poor growth.

* Double-check your schedule. You should allow two to three hours between meals and snacks to allow your child to develop an appetite.

* Only offer water to drink between meals since milk between meals can impact your child's appetite.

  * Serve milk in an open cup—this can slow down the process of drinking and help bring your child's attention back to their food.

  * If your child drinks their milk when a meal is presented, then asks for more milk rather than eating their food, serve the milk immediately after the meal so they'll satisfy their hunger with food first.

YOUR CHILD REFUSES FOOD PREVIOUSLY ENJOYED: Sometime between 12 to 18 months of age, children hit a phase called *food neophobia*. The theory behind why this phase occurs is that as children start walking, they could wander outside and pick something poisonous off the ground. To coincide with this newfound freedom, they develop a newfound fear of foods. This phase does end, but in the meantime, continue to offer your child a variety of foods, enjoy them together, always include a familiar food item that they have continued to accept, and refrain from encouraging or pushing them. Once you have set the food down in front of your child, your job is to sit together and not to return to the kitchen to make something else for them. See chapter 6 (page 154) for more detailed tips on working through this selective phase.

QUINOA BOWL

GLUTEN-FREE **NUT-FREE OPTION** VEGETARIAN VEGAN OPTION

YIELDS 3 SERVINGS

1 cup cooked quinoa

1 cup milk or full-fat plain Greek yogurt (yogurt or milk alternative for vegan option)

1 cup berries

¼ cup toppings (shelled hemp seeds, sunflower seeds, finely chopped nuts, shredded coconut)

Quinoa is often considered a rice replacement or an enjoyable addition to a salad. We use it in the Quinoa Pizza Bites (page 49), but quinoa in a parfait may be new territory. This recipe takes your yogurt parfait and rounds it out for lasting satisfaction. Serve this snack deconstructed so family members can create their own perfect bowls.

1. Separate the ingredients into serving bowls and place them on the table with serving spoons.

2. Have each family member build a bowl, using quinoa as a base.

TO REFRIGERATE: Store in a sealed container and refrigerate the assembled bowl for up to 2 days.

MORNING GLORY MUFFINS

NUT-FREE VEGAN

YIELDS 18 MUFFINS

Nonstick cooking spray (optional)

1½ cups whole-wheat flour

½ cup all-purpose flour

¾ cup brown sugar

1 tablespoon baking powder

2 teaspoons baking soda

2 teaspoons cinnamon

½ teaspoon salt

¾ cup applesauce

½ cup coconut oil or butter, melted

1 apple, grated

1 tablespoon vanilla extract

2 cups carrot, grated

½ cup raisins

Muffins are a staple in my house. They're nutritious, they're freezable, and they defrost quickly. These muffins are perfect for little hands and make a great snack. You can make a double batch and fill your freezer for those unexpected busy days. Like the Chocolate Bloomies (page 76) batter, this dough is thick because the shredded carrots and apples release moisture as they bake.

1. Preheat the oven to 375°F.

2. Prepare two 12-cup muffin tins with paper or silicone liners or grease the pan with the nonstick cooking spray, if using.

3. Mix the flours, sugar, baking powder, baking soda, cinnamon, and salt in a large mixing bowl.

4. In a medium-size mixing bowl, combine the applesauce, oil, apple, and vanilla.

5. Pour the wet ingredients into the dry ingredients and mix until just combined.

6. Fold in the carrots and raisins.

7. Fill each muffin cup to two-thirds full and bake for 25 to 28 minutes, or until golden.

CHANGE IT UP:

- To increase the flavor, try adding ½ teaspoon of ground ginger in step 3.
- To increase the protein and crunch, fold in ½ cup of chopped walnuts in step 6.
- To increase the texture, add ½ cup of shredded (desiccated) coconut in step 6 or top the muffins with it just before baking.

TO REFRIGERATE: Store in a sealed container or bag for 3 to 5 days.

TO FREEZE: Place in a freezer-safe bag, remove all air, and freeze for up to 4 months.

PLANTAIN TOSTONES

GLUTEN-FREE **NUT FREE** VEGAN

YIELDS 6 SERVINGS

2 green plantains

¼ cup rice flour

½ cup cooking oil, like avocado oil

Sea salt

TO REFRIGERATE:
Cover and store in a sealed container for up to 3 days.

CHANGE IT UP:
If plantains are not available in your area, consider substituting bananas. I love Burro, red, and even baby bananas for this recipe. Rice flour can be substituted with all-purpose flour.

Some of the best and most delicious foods are the simplest recipes. Tostones contain Caribbean and Latin American flavors, and they're often consumed as a street food snack in those regions. Cutting these into half-inch chunks makes them smaller for tiny hands to enjoy. It is essential to fry these treats twice. The first fry releases the starches in the plantain but doesn't soften the texture. The second fry at a higher temperature steams then softens the inside while giving the outside a crispy crunch. You can enjoy these tostones hot or cold.

1. Peel the plantains. Slice off the top and bottom of the plantain with a sharp knife. Slice lengthwise through the tough outer skin in three places. Peel the skin from the plantain to expose the starchy fruit. Discard the skins.

2. Slice the plantains into discs about ½ inch thick. Dust each disc in rice flour.

3. Heat the oil in a nonstick skillet on medium heat. Fry the plantains for 2 to 3 minutes on each side. Drain excess oil on a kitchen towel.

4. Place the fried plantain discs on a sheet of parchment paper. Sprinkle them with rice flour, then cover with another sheet of parchment paper. Roll or mash the plantains gently between the parchment paper.

5. Increase the temperature for the skillet to medium-high heat. Fry the plantains for 2 to 3 minutes on each side, until golden brown.

6. Drain on a kitchen towel and sprinkle immediately with sea salt.

DIPPED BANANA AND CHIA JAM SANDWICH

GLUTEN-FREE **NUT-FREE** VEGETARIAN VEGAN OPTION

**YIELDS 5
SANDWICHES**

1 pound fresh
strawberries,
(or frozen and
thawed), hulled and
roughly chopped

3 tablespoons honey
or maple syrup

1 teaspoon
lemon juice

2 tablespoons
chia seeds

1 banana

½ cup plain full-fat
Greek yogurt (yogurt
alternative for
vegan option)

These sandwiches are a great snack or side. They have a tart bite that is mellowed by the sweetness of the banana. Once you get rolling with chia jam, you can break out of the mold and try different flavors. I love to make it with berries and a squeeze of lemon, but the options are endless. You can use the remaining chia jam for PB&J Sandwich Kabobs (page 107), French Toast Sticks (page 78), or even as an oatmeal mix-in (page 31).

1. In a medium pot over medium heat, boil the chopped strawberries and honey. The strawberries will release moisture and then begin to boil.

2. As bubbles begin to form, remove from heat and use a metal fork or a potato masher to carefully mash the hot strawberries.

3. Mix in the lemon juice and the chia seeds, then let the mixture sit, uncovered, to cool.

4. When the chia jam has reached room temperature to slightly warm, peel the banana and slice it into 10 slices.

5. Prepare a baking sheet by lining it with parchment paper or foil. Place the banana slices on the prepared baking sheet.

CONTINUED

6. Cover a banana slice with some chia jam, then top it with another banana slice to make a sandwich.

7. Make 5 sandwiches, then set aside the remaining chia jam.

8. Freeze the sandwiches for 45 to 60 minutes.

9. Take the sandwiches out of the freezer and dip them, either half or whole, in the yogurt. Place them back on the pan and freeze for at least an hour.

10. Enjoy!

CHANGE IT UP:
Try making chia jam with blueberries, raspberries, blackberries, mixed berries, peaches, or other stone fruits.

FROZEN YOGURT BARK

GLUTEN-FREE **NUT-FREE OPTION** VEGETARIAN VEGAN OPTION

YIELDS 6 SERVINGS

2 cups full-fat Greek yogurt (yogurt alternative for vegan option)

2 tablespoons maple syrup

½ teaspoon vanilla extract

½ cup toppings (sliced strawberries, blueberries, shredded coconut, dark chocolate shavings, finely chopped dried cranberries or raisins, crushed nuts, hulled hemp seeds, ½ teaspoon lemon zest)

Yogurt is full of delicious health benefits. The fat is great for brain growth and development. The probiotics are wonderful for gut health. I like to suggest Greek yogurt because it has more protein and calcium than regular yogurt. And it is such a versatile food. This colorful dish could double as a snack or dessert, and even the tiniest hands can help create it. Set out some topping options, spread out your yogurt, and let your little one help sprinkle colorful goodness on your treat.

1. Mix the yogurt, maple syrup, and vanilla extract in a small mixing bowl.

2. Line a baking tray with wax paper.

3. Pour the yogurt mix onto the prepared baking tray and spread it evenly, ideally not thicker than ½ inch at any point.

4. Sprinkle the toppings over the yogurt.

5. Place in the freezer for 2 to 4 hours, until hard, then use a sharp knife to break the bark into pieces. Enjoy!

TO FREEZE: Store the cut pieces in a freezer-safe bag or airtight container for up to 1 month.

SWEET POTATO WAFFLES

GLUTEN-FREE OPTION **NUT-FREE** VEGETARIAN VEGAN OPTION

**YIELDS 11 TO
12 WAFFLES**

2 cups all-purpose
flour (gluten-free flour
optional)

¼ teaspoon sea salt

1 tablespoon double-
acting baking powder

3 large eggs (flax eggs
for vegan option)

½ cup milk (milk
alternative for
vegan option)

½ cup buttermilk
(buttermilk
alternative for
vegan option)

½ cup melted butter
(butter alternative for
vegan option)

1 teaspoon
vanilla extract

1 tablespoon
maple syrup

1 cup sweet
potato purée

Airy waffles that are so sweet they don't need syrup? Yes, please! The trick to light and airy waffles is to not overmix the batter. Mixing too much will give the waffle a firm texture and make it dense. Allow the batter to rest for 5 minutes after mixing while your waffle iron heats. The waffles will expand in the iron, so remember that a little batter goes a long way.

1. Combine the flour, salt, and baking powder in a small bowl and whisk to mix.

2. In a large bowl, whisk the eggs. Add the milk and buttermilk and whisk. Add the melted butter and mix well. Add the vanilla, maple syrup, and sweet potato, mixing well.

3. Add the flour mixture to the wet ingredients, folding gently to incorporate, making sure not to overmix.

4. Let the batter rest for 5 minutes to activate the baking powder.

5. Preheat the waffle iron.

6. Spoon the batter into the preheated waffle iron.

7. Cook for 5 to 7 minutes according to your waffle iron instructions.

COOKING TIP:
- This recipe works well with nondairy milk and butter sources.
- To make buttermilk, mix 1 teaspoon of lemon juice with 1 cup of milk.

CHANGE IT UP: Include 1 teaspoon of pumpkin pie spice, which pairs deliciously with sweet potatoes.

TO STORE: Refrigeration tends to dry out the trapped moisture and can leave these waffles tasting stale. Store at room temperature for up to 1 day and reheat in a toaster or oven.

TO FREEZE: Place cooled waffles between a section of folded parchment paper and freeze flat in an airtight container. Toast from frozen and enjoy hot.

KEDGEREE WITH FLAKED WHITEFISH

GLUTEN-FREE **NUT-FREE**

YIELDS 4 (1-CUP) SERVINGS

1 cup long grain rice

1½ cups water

4 large eggs

2 tablespoons olive oil

½ Vidalia onion, diced

2 garlic cloves, minced

1 tablespoon curry powder

2 teaspoons salt

1 cup heavy cream

2½ pounds whitefish, like smoked haddock

1 bay leaf

1 tablespoon lemon juice

½ cup minced flat leaf parsley

This flavorful dish is usually served for breakfast, but it also makes a delicious lunch or dinner. Gently simmering the rice in the flavored cream softens the rice and deepens the flavors.

1. Rinse the rice under cold water until the water runs clear. Pour 1½ cups of water into a pot and add the rice. Bring to a boil, then reduce heat to low, cooking for 10 minutes. Check for doneness (see tip), then drain and discard any remaining cooking water. Set the rice aside.

2. In the same pot, bring salted water to a boil and cook the eggs for 10 minutes. When the eggs are finished cooking, immerse them immediately in ice water to stop them from cooking further.

3. When the eggs are cool, peel and chop them, then set aside.

4. Heat the olive oil on medium in a clean pot. When the oil shimmers and quickly coats the bottom, add the onion and garlic and sauté until translucent, careful to avoid burning. Add the curry powder and sauté for 1 minute. Add the salt, heavy cream, fish, and bay leaf.

5. Bring to a simmer. Remove the bay leaf, add the rice and lemon juice, and mix to coat with sauce. Cook for 5 minutes.

6. Remove the pot from the heat and add the parsley and chopped eggs. Gently fold to mix.

COOKING TIP: To determine if the rice is cooked, taste it. If it's chewy or hard in the center, then add ⅛ to ¼ cup of water, place the lid on the pot, and cook the rice for another 3 to 5 minutes on very low heat.

CHANGE IT UP: Haddock and pollack are generally found in the freezer section of your local grocery store and make a great affordable dish in place of smoked haddock.

SAFETY TIP: Babies and children up to age six should not eat fish that is known to have high levels of mercury. Avoid fresh or frozen tuna, shark, swordfish, marlin, orange roughy, and canned albacore tuna.

TO REFRIGERATE: Store in a sealed container for up to 3 days.

TO FREEZE: Freeze in an airtight container for up to 2 months. Defrost overnight in the refrigerator, then gently reheat covered in the microwave

CORNBREAD WITH SCRAMBLED EGGS

GLUTEN-FREE OPTION **NUT-FREE** VEGETARIAN

YIELDS 4 SERVINGS

FOR THE CORNBREAD

2½ cups yellow cornmeal

1 cup all-purpose flour (gluten-free flour optional)

2 teaspoons salt

1 teaspoon baking powder

1 teaspoon baking soda

2 large eggs

1 cup milk

1¾ cups buttermilk

2 tablespoons melted butter

FOR THE SCRAMBLED EGGS

4 large eggs

¼ cup milk

Pinch salt

Pinch pepper

2 teaspoons butter

The flavorful pairing of savory scrambled eggs and skillet cornbread is sure to be a family favorite. This recipe bakes best in a cast iron skillet, but it stays moist in a loaf or pie pan. Traditional southern cornbread gets all its sweetness from the sweet yellow cornmeal, so no additional sugar is needed. The soft-texture pairing of eggs and cornbread makes for a great baby-led weaning option. If you don't have buttermilk, see page 127 for a homemade version.

TO MAKE THE CORNBREAD

1. Preheat a cast iron skillet in the oven at 375°F.

2. In a mixing bowl, whisk together the cornmeal, flour, salt, baking powder, and baking soda.

3. In a separate bowl, whisk together the eggs, milk, buttermilk, and melted butter.

4. Add the dry ingredients to the wet ingredients, then fold to incorporate.

5. Add the batter to the hot skillet, smoothing the top with a spatula. Bake for 35 minutes, or until a toothpick inserted in the center comes out clean.

6. Cool in the pan on a wire rack. Slice and serve hot.

1. In a medium-size mixing bowl, beat the eggs, milk, salt, and pepper.

2. Heat the butter in a large pan over medium heat until it just begins to brown.

3. Pour the egg mixture into the pan. As the eggs begin to set, use a spatula to pull them apart and form large, soft pieces.

4. Continue cooking by pulling, lifting, and folding the eggs until no liquid egg remains.

5. Serve after cooling to warm.

CHANGE IT UP:

- This recipe works well with nondairy milk and butter sources.
- For the cornbread, at step 2, add ½ cup of frozen corn or a seeded, diced jalapeño for a southwestern take on a traditional favorite.

TO STORE: Store cornbread in an airtight container at room temperature. Do not refrigerate; the cornbread will get stale faster in the refrigerator. Eggs should be made fresh, as they do not store well in the refrigerator or freezer.

TO FREEZE: Slice the cornbread, then freeze in an airtight container for up to 2 months.

EGG AND CHEESE BREAKFAST QUESADILLA

GLUTEN-FREE **NUT-FREE** **VEGETARIAN**

**YIELDS 4
QUESADILLAS**

2 tablespoons
butter, divided into
4 equal pieces

4 large eggs

8 corn
tortillas, warmed

2 cups shredded
Mexican cheese

This quesadilla is simple and straightforward with few ingredients. The quesadillas freeze remarkably well and are easy to reheat on a busy morning.

1. In a skillet over medium heat, melt 1 piece of butter. Crack 1 egg into the skillet. Use a spatula to break the yolk, cook for 1 minute, then flip. Cook on the other side for 1 minute. Remove from the skillet and set aside. Repeat with remaining eggs.

2. Place 1 warmed tortilla to cook in the same skillet.

3. Top the tortilla with shredded cheese. Add a cooked egg and top with more cheese. Top with a second tortilla.

4. Cover and let cook for 1 minute.

5. Flip and cook covered on the other side for 1 minute.

6. Repeat steps 2 through 5 the with remaining tortillas.

7. Cut each quesadilla in half, then in half again. Serve hot with your favorite salsa.

TO REFRIGERATE: Allow to cool completely, then layer between parchment paper in an airtight container. Refrigerate for no more than 3 days.

TO FREEZE: Store in an airtight container with parchment paper between layers. Freeze for up to 3 months.

CREPES WITH HAZELNUT SPREAD

GLUTEN-FREE **VEGETARIAN**

YIELDS 8 CREPES

¼ cup milk

3 large eggs

1 teaspoon
vanilla extract

½ cup tapioca flour

Pinch salt

4 tablespoons butter,
divided into 8 pieces

1 jar hazelnut
spread, warmed

1 cup strawberries,
hulled and
thinly sliced

CHANGE IT UP: Fill crepes with lemon curd and whipped cream, cashew butter and sliced bananas, or my personal favorite, warmed marionberry jam and a dollop of whipped cream.

Crepes are delicate and airy French pancakes. The trick is to have your butter portioned and a measuring cup for the batter ready. From there, it just takes a swirl of the wrist to spread the batter out thinly. I use a regular 10-inch shallow skillet and a silicone spatula, so there's no need to buy a crepe pan. Serve these as sweet crepes for brunch or a decadent afternoon snack. Prefer to have a savory crepe? Omit the vanilla and top with meats, cheeses, or eggs. My favorite hazelnut spread is Justin's Chocolate Hazelnut and Almond Butter.

1. In a small bowl, whisk the milk with the eggs until smooth. Add the vanilla and whisk to mix.

2. In a medium bowl, mix the tapioca flour and salt.

3. Add the wet ingredients to the dry mixture and stir gently to mix. The batter will be runny.

4. Heat 1 piece of butter in a 10-inch nonstick skillet over medium heat.

5. Add ¼ cup of batter to the pan and swirl to coat. Cook for 30 to 50 seconds.

CONTINUED

BREAKFAST

6. Gently flip the crepe with a spatula and cook for 30 to 50 seconds more.

7. Place the crepe on a kitchen towel and cover to keep warm as you cook the remaining crepes.

8. To serve, spread the warmed hazelnut spread across the crepe. Top with the strawberries.

TO REFRIGERATE: Allow the crepes to cool completely, then layer them between parchment paper in an airtight container. Refrigerate for no more than 3 days.

TO FREEZE: Freeze crepes prior to filling. Store in an airtight, sealed container, such as a freezer-safe zip-top bag. Defrost overnight in the refrigerator and reheat, covered, from refrigerated for 30 seconds in the microwave.

COOKING TIP: Traditional crepes are made with buckwheat, which has a very strong flavor. Tapioca is milder and works well in this recipe. Traditional all-purpose flour mixed with 1 teaspoon of cornstarch makes a great pastry flour for this recipe. Be sure to sift your pastry flour to prevent lumps from forming in the batter.

ACAI FRUIT BOWL

GLUTEN-FREE **NUT-FREE** VEGAN

YIELDS 2 (1-CUP) SERVINGS

8 ounces acai juice

1 banana, diced into chunks, frozen

½ cup pitted cherries, frozen

Toppings of choice

CHANGE IT UP: Instead of acai and cherries, try frozen peach chunks and peach nectar; frozen raspberries, strawberries, and 2 tablespoons of lime juice; or frozen mango or pineapple chunks and 8 ounces of coconut milk.

This naturally super sweet recipe is a decadent breakfast or afternoon treat on a hot day. Born out of a trip to Brazil, these delicious bowls can be served in the early afternoon for a cooling escape from the summer heat. Slice and freeze your bananas to make fruit bowls easy to make. Acai (ah-sa-YEE) juice or purée can be used for this recipe. The juice is more widely available, but the purée can be found in the freezer section of some grocery stores. If you're not able to find any acai, you can substitute pomegranate juice. This recipe is a favorite for teething babies and those with sore throats.

1. Combine the acai juice, banana, and cherries in a blender.

2. Blend until smooth.

3. Add toppings of choice such as frozen berries, granola, almond slivers, or diced chocolate.

TO FREEZE: Fruit can be frozen in 4- or 8-ounce portions. Thaw frozen fruit or juice prior to blending.

BABY-LED FEEDING TIP: Leave this smoothie bowl coarsely blended to add texture for a baby-led feeding food. Provide your child with a loaded spoon and watch them go!

FLATBREAD PIZZA

GLUTEN-FREE OPTION **NUT-FREE** VEGETARIAN VEGAN OPTION

YIELDS 4 SERVINGS

Vegetables for topping, such as spinach, bell peppers, mushrooms, cherry tomatoes (halved lengthwise)

Olive oil spray (optional)

1 flatbread (gluten-free flatbread optional)

3 tablespoons marinara sauce, Veggieful Sauce (page 73), or pesto

2 ounces shredded mozzarella cheese (cheese alternative for vegan option)

¼ teaspoon Italian seasoning

Who doesn't love a good pizza? Flatbread pizza can make a quick dinner, or a do-it-yourself pizza party. Pizza is a wonderful canvas for colorful veggies and can be a great way to gently expose your child to more colors in food. Start with a great flatbread—lavash, tortillas, or matzo work well—and build a masterpiece together.

1. Preheat the oven to 450°F.

2. Chop the vegetables for topping and set aside.

3. Prepare a baking sheet by spraying it with oil or lining it with a sheet of parchment paper. Lay out the flatbread on the prepared pan.

4. Spread the sauce on the flatbread with a spoon, being careful not to add too much, or the flatbread will become soggy.

5. Add the vegetables and sprinkle the cheese and Italian seasoning on top.

6. Bake until the cheese is melted and starts to brown, 10 to 15 minutes.

7. Let cool, slice, and enjoy!

TO REFRIGERATE: Place the flatbread on a tray in a single layer and cover tightly. Keep for up to a day and reheat in the oven or enjoy cold.

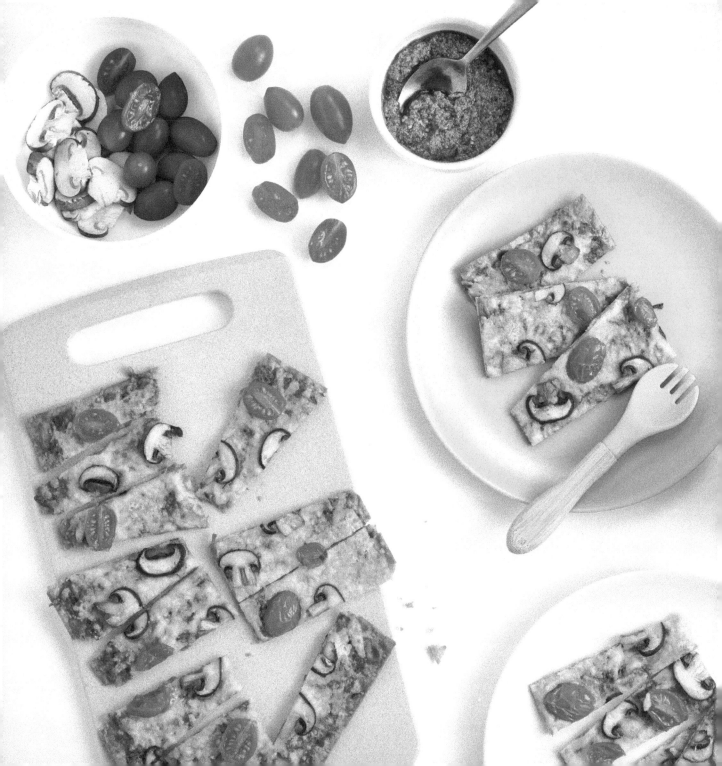

SOUTHWESTERN QUINOA SALAD

GLUTEN-FREE **NUT-FREE** VEGAN

YIELDS 8 SERVINGS

3 cups cooked quinoa

1 large bell
pepper, diced

11 ounces fresh or
frozen corn niblets

1 (15-ounce) can
black beans, drained
and rinsed

4 green onions, sliced

⅓ cup olive oil

2 teaspoons lime zest

½ cup lime juice

1 teaspoon
kosher salt

Black pepper

Quinoa comes in different colors. A mixed color option is my personal favorite, but any color can be used in this recipe. White quinoa is lighter, and the red and black versions are heartier. Mix this salad up for your family or take it to the next potluck party. It's always a hit.

In a large mixing bowl, stir together the quinoa, bell pepper, corn, black beans, green onions, olive oil, lime zest, lime juice, salt, and pepper. Serve.

TO REFRIGERATE: Store in a sealed container for up to 3 days.

CHANGE IT UP: Add ¼ cup of chopped fresh cilantro or 1 cubed avocado for a great flavor boost.

EGG SALAD LETTUCE CUPS

GLUTEN-FREE **NUT-FREE** VEGETARIAN

YIELDS 4 TO 6 SERVINGS

1 head butter
leaf lettuce

6 large eggs, room
temperature

1½ teaspoons
salt, divided

¼ cup finely chopped
red onion

1 tablespoon minced
fresh parsley

1 celery stalk, diced

¼ cup mayonnaise

2 teaspoons mustard

1 teaspoon
lemon juice

½ teaspoon
ground pepper

Egg salad is easy to eat and soft for your weaning baby who's exploring new foods. Have your little one help with peeling and mashing the eggs (under close supervision). The tender, open leaves of butter leaf lettuce will invite your little one for a taste.

1. Wash the lettuce from the top of the leaves, running the water through to the bottom stalk. Stand the leaves upright on the stalk to dry. When dry, cut and discard the stalk.

2. Place the eggs in a pot and cover with warm water. Add 1 teaspoon of salt. Bring to a boil over high heat, then reduce the heat to medium-high. Cook for 10 minutes. Drain the eggs, then plunge them into ice water to halt cooking.

3. Peel and rinse the eggs, then chop into small chunks. When the eggs are cool, toss them with the red onion, parsley, and celery.

4. In a small bowl, to make the sauce, whisk together the mayonnaise, mustard, lemon juice, pepper, and the remaining ½ teaspoon of salt.

5. Add the sauce to the egg mixture and fold gently to incorporate.

6. Spoon the egg mixture into the lettuce cups and serve warm.

TO REFRIGERATE: Store in an airtight container for up to 5 days.

MINESTRONE SOUP

GLUTEN-FREE OPTION **NUT-FREE** VEGAN

YIELDS 4 (2-CUP) SERVINGS

1 tablespoon olive oil

1 onion, diced

3 garlic cloves, minced

2 carrots, peeled and cut into coins

1 tablespoon Italian seasoning

1 medium zucchini, cut into bite-size chunks

2 cups Swiss chard, trimmed

1 (32-ounce) box low-sodium vegetable broth

1 (15-ounce) can cannellini beans, drained and rinsed

1 (15-ounce) can diced tomatoes

1 cup pasta, cooked according to package instructions (gluten-free pasta optional)

This easy-to-prepare soup is filled with the delicious vegetables of early fall. Cutting the vegetables into small bites is key for maximum toddler enjoyment. Enhance the soup's flavor by topping it with a spoonful of pesto and a sprinkle of shredded Parmesan cheese.

1. In a 4-quart stockpot over medium heat, heat the oil. Sauté the onion and garlic in the oil for 2 minutes.

2. Add the carrots and Italian seasoning. Sauté for 2 minutes.

3. Add the zucchini and chard. Sauté for 1 minute.

4. Add the broth. Cook for 6 minutes on medium heat, until the soup just starts to boil, then reduce the heat to low to simmer.

5. Add the beans and tomatoes with their juice and simmer for 3 minutes.

6. Divide the pasta into four bowls.

7. Serve the soup hot, over pasta.

TO REFRIGERATE: Store in a sealed container for up to 5 days.

TO FREEZE: Store in an airtight container for up to 2 months. Defrost overnight in the refrigerator. Gently warm in a saucepan over medium heat.

CHANGE IT UP:

• Substitute chard with spinach and add at step 5.

• Consider adding 2 cups of trimmed kale at step 5 for added vitamins and flavor.

CHICKEN, BACON, AVOCADO, AND RANCH PASTA

GLUTEN-FREE OPTION **NUT-FREE**

YIELDS 4 (1-CUP) SERVINGS

1 avocado, peeled and pitted

1 (1-ounce) ranch dressing dry mix packet

1 cup Alfredo sauce

2 tablespoons minced fresh parsley

½ tablespoon cooking oil

2 garlic cloves, minced

1 shallot, finely diced

2 cups boneless, skinless diced chicken breasts or thighs

Pinch salt

Pinch pepper

4 strips bacon, thinly sliced

8 ounces pasta, cooked according to package instructions (gluten-free pasta optional)

Children love pasta, and it's easy to eat with their hands as they learn to feed themselves. Use small tubular pastas like penne or mostaccioli. Using a premade Alfredo sauce speeds up the prep and cook time, and the cool ranch flavor is balanced by the subtle creaminess of the avocado.

1. In a mixing bowl, combine the avocado, ranch dressing mix, Alfredo sauce, and parsley. Whisk well.

2. Heat the cooking oil in a shallow pan over medium heat. Sauté the garlic and shallot for 2 minutes. Add the chicken, salt, and pepper, and cook until browned, 5 to 7 minutes.

3. Add the bacon and cook until crispy.

4. Add the ranch mixture and cooked pasta, stirring to coat.

5. Simmer the mixture for 3 minutes.

6. Serve warm to hot.

TO REFRIGERATE: Store in a sealed container for up to 3 days. Reheat in the microwave or bake at 350°F for up to 15 minutes, or until hot.

CHANGE IT UP: Sun-dried tomatoes are a delicious addition.

SAVORY SWEET POTATO GNOCCHI

GLUTEN-FREE OPTION **NUT-FREE** VEGETARIAN

YIELDS 4 (1-CUP) SERVINGS

2 cups canned sweet potatoes

2 teaspoons salt

3 garlic cloves, minced, divided

1 large egg, beaten, room temperature

2½ cups all-purpose flour (gluten-free flour optional), divided

2 tablespoons butter

1 tablespoon olive oil

2 cups spinach, trimmed

½ cup Parmesan cheese, divided

These gnocchi are easy to make and so delicious. The most important step is to strain the sweet potatoes. Removing the extra moisture is key to bringing the dough together.

1. Strain the potatoes in a cheesecloth and reserve the liquid.

2. In a medium bowl, season the potatoes with the salt and 1 clove of minced garlic. Make a small well in the center of the potatoes. Add the beaten egg to the well and mix with a silicone spatula.

3. Add 2 cups of flour, ½ cup at a time, mixing between additions until almost incorporated. A soft dough should start to form.

4. Turn the contents of the bowl onto a clean counter or cutting board. Knead the dough gently to fully incorporate the flour, being careful not to overmix. The dough should be smooth and silky, not sticky.

5. Section the dough into 6 pieces. Working from the center toward the outside, roll each piece into a log shape about 6 inches long. Cut each log into 1-inch pieces and toss in the remaining ½ cup flour. Roll each piece down the back of a fork or across a ridged pasta board.

6. Fill a pot with salted water. Allow the gnocchi to rest for 15 minutes while the water comes to a boil.

7. Test one or two gnocchi before boiling all the pasta. If the gnocchi hold their shape, the dough has enough flour and the remaining gnocchi can be cooked. If the gnocchi fall apart in the water, add more flour to the dough, 1 tablespoon at a time, until the gnocchi hold their shape when boiled.

8. Boil the gnocchi in batches for 5 to 7 minutes, or until they float. Remove with a slotted spoon.

9. In a sauté pan, heat the butter and olive oil over medium heat. When the butter foams, add the remaining 2 cloves of minced garlic. Sauté for 1 minute, until fragrant. Add the cooked gnocchi and reserved sweet potato liquid. Cook for 2 minutes. Add the spinach and ¼ cup of Parmesan cheese. Sauté for 1 minute.

10. Remove the pan from heat. Garnish the gnocchi with the remaining ¼ cup of Parmesan cheese. Serve hot.

TO REFRIGERATE: Store in an airtight container for up to 3 days.

TO FREEZE: Stop after step 5 and store in an airtight container. Cook from frozen in salted boiling water.

BLACK BEAN BURRITO BOWL WITH MANGO AND AVOCADO SALSA

GLUTEN-FREE **NUT-FREE** VEGAN OPTION

YIELDS 6 (1-CUP) SERVINGS

FOR THE DRESSING

3 tablespoons lime juice

1 tablespoon olive oil

2 tablespoons chopped cilantro

½ teaspoon canned chipotle chiles

¼ teaspoon ground black pepper

¼ teaspoon salt

FOR THE BURRITO BOWL

1 head romaine lettuce

1 tablespoon cooking oil

1 garlic clove, minced

1 teaspoon diced shallot

½ cup low-sodium vegetable or chicken broth

Although this flavorful Black Bean Burrito Bowl has many ingredients, it is quick and easy to make. Consider topping it with grilled chicken, shrimp, or beef flank steak, or add some tortilla strips for a crispy crunch. Be sure to include some Guacamole (page 161) on the side! Any leftovers can be used in Black Bean, Chicken, and Corn Arepas (page 148).

TO MAKE THE DRESSING

Blend the lime juice, olive oil, cilantro, chiles, pepper, and salt in a blender until smooth.

TO MAKE THE BURRITO BOWL

1. Wash the romaine lettuce, running the water from the top of the leaves through to the bottom stalk. Stand upright on the stalk to dry. When dry, cut and discard the stalk. Shred the lettuce into bite-size pieces.

2. Toss the lettuce in the dressing and portion to serve.

3. In a medium saucepan, heat the cooking oil over medium heat. Add the garlic and shallot and cook for 1 minute. Add the broth and bring to a simmer.

4. Add the black beans, cover, and steam for 5 minutes. Drain.

5. Top the lettuce with the black beans and steamed corn.

TO MAKE THE SALSA

1. Combine the avocado, mangos, onion, bell pepper, tomato, jalapeño, and jicama in a medium bowl, tossing with a fork to mix.

2. Top the burrito bowl with the salsa.

CHANGE IT UP: Pinto beans also work well in this recipe and can substitute for black beans.

SAFETY TIP: Be sure to wash the cilantro well before use.

FOR THE BURRITO BOWL continued

1 (15-ounce) can black beans, drained and rinsed

15 ounces frozen or canned corn, steamed

FOR THE SALSA

1 large avocado, peeled, pitted, and diced into cubes

2 mangos, peeled, pitted, and diced

½ sweet onion, diced

1 red bell pepper, diced

1 tomato, diced

1 jalapeño, seeded and diced

1 cup diced jicama

MACARONI AND CHEESE CUPS

GLUTEN-FREE OPTION **NUT-FREE** **VEGETARIAN**

YIELDS 12
MUFFIN CUPS

½ cup bread crumbs
(gluten-free bread
crumbs optional)

1 tablespoon
butter, melted

1 garlic clove, minced

1 tablespoon
chopped fresh parsley

4 cups
shredded cheese

4 tablespoons all-
purpose flour (gluten-
free flour optional)

¼ teaspoon salt

Pinch black pepper

1 cup heavy cream

1 cup milk

¼ teaspoon
dry mustard

8 ounces elbow
macaroni, cooked al
dente (gluten-free
pasta optional)

This is the ultimate comfort food in small muffin-size portions. These cups
are perfectly sized to pack for lunch for your preschooler or for using for
baby-led feeding. I prefer silicone liners for this recipe, since they hold
their shape well at high temperatures and prevent excessive drying.

1. Preheat the oven to 375°F.

2. In a small bowl, combine the bread crumbs, melted butter, garlic,
and parsley. Set aside.

3. In a medium bowl, combine the cheese, flour, salt, and pepper,
tossing to mix.

4. In a medium saucepan, bring the cream, milk, and mustard to a
gentle boil, stirring often.

5. Add the cheese mixture to the cream mixture. Mix well and cook
until the cheese is melted and the mixture is bubbly.

6. Remove the saucepan from the heat, then add the cooked macaroni to the cheese sauce. Stir to mix and let rest for 5 minutes.

7. Place silicone liners into a muffin tin. Spoon the macaroni mixture into the muffin cups and top with the bread crumb mixture.

8. Bake the cups for 10 to 15 minutes, or until cheese sauce is bubbly and the bread crumbs are browned.

TO REFRIGERATE: Store in an airtight container for up to 5 days.

TO FREEZE: Store in an airtight container for up to 2 months.

COOKING TIP: Pea protein milk or rice milk makes a great nondairy substitution for the milk, while cashew cream is a good substitution for the heavy cream. Other nut milks are often sweetened and can alter the flavor of the sauce.

BLACK BEAN, CHICKEN, AND CORN AREPAS

GLUTEN-FREE **NUT-FREE** VEGETARIAN OPTION VEGAN OPTION

YIELDS 8 AREPAS

FOR THE FILLING

2 pounds boneless, skinless chicken breasts or thighs, diced (alternative for vegetarian or vegan option)

1 teaspoon salt

½ teaspoon black pepper

1 teaspoon garlic powder

1 tablespoon avocado oil

1 garlic clove, minced

1 teaspoon diced shallot

½ cup low-sodium vegetable or chicken broth

1 (15-ounce) can black beans, drained and rinsed

15 ounces frozen corn niblets

This recipe uses many of the same ingredients as the Black Bean Burrito Bowl (page 144) and makes a great follow-up recipe if you want to use up any leftovers you have from making those bowls. An arepa is a cross between a tortilla and a pancake. Arepas are a staple in South America and very versatile. You can make them small—perfect for tiny hands. Seeking a vegetarian or vegan option? Substitute your favorite alternative meat and milk for the chicken and milk in this recipe. Make it a meal by serving the arepas with Plantain Tostones (page 122).

TO MAKE THE FILLING

1. Season the chicken with the salt, pepper, and garlic powder.

2. In a skillet over medium heat, heat the avocado oil. Add the garlic and shallot and cook for 1 minute. Add the chicken and cook for 5 to 7 minutes, or until browned.

3. Add the broth and bring to a simmer. Add the black beans. Steam for 5 minutes.

4. Add the corn and cook for 1 minute. Remove the skillet from the heat and allow the mixture to cool.

TO MAKE THE AREPAS

1. In a bowl, combine the Sweet Corn Mix, water, and milk to form a soft dough. Divide the dough into 8 equal portions and press each

into the palm of your hand, flattening it out and creating a lip around the edge.

2. Spoon some of the chicken filling into the center of an arepa. Work the edges back toward the center to enclose the filling inside. Repeat for the remaining arepas.

3. Allow the arepas to rest for 3 minutes. Heat the cooking oil in a shallow pan over medium-high heat.

4. Cook each arepa for about 3 minutes on each side, or until lightly browned.

5. Serve with Guacamole (page 161) or Mango and Avocado Salsa (page 145).

TO FREEZE: Follow the cooling and packaging instructions for refrigerating. Freeze for up to 2 months.

COOKING TIP: The PAN mix has been precooked and dried with added sugar, rice flour, salt, and xanthan gum. If it is not available in your area, you can order it online, or you can use your favorite cornbread mix instead.

CHANGE IT UP: Fill these arepas with your favorite food combinations: chicken, cheese, and frozen vegetables; Beef and Pumpkin Purée (page 63); chicken, bacon, and avocado; pulled pork, corn, and cheese; shredded beef, onion, and grilled diced peppers; or pineapple, corn, and cheese.

FOR THE AREPAS

1½ cups PAN Sweet Corn Mix

1 cup water

¼ cup milk (milk alternative for vegan option)

2 tablespoons cooking oil

TO REFRIGERATE: Allow the arepas to cool to room temperature and place a piece of parchment paper between them. Store in the refrigerator for up to 5 days.

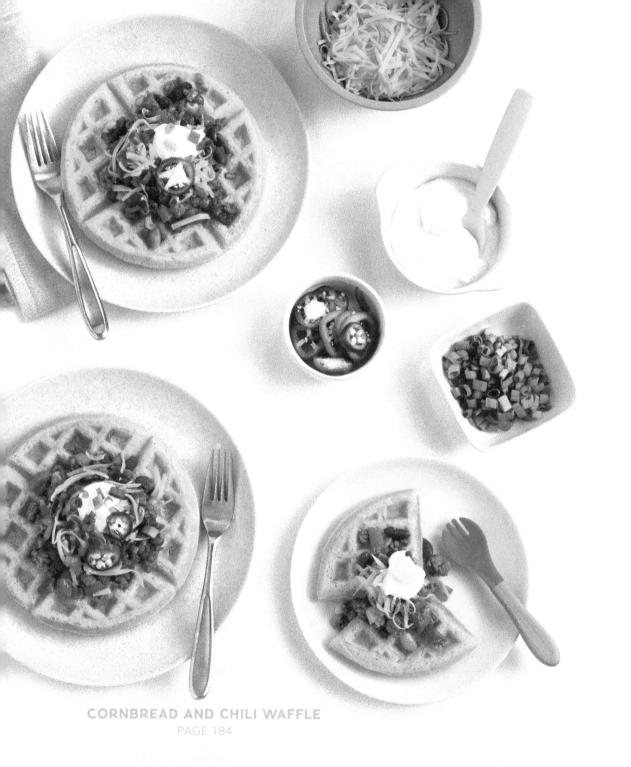

CORNBREAD AND CHILI WAFFLE
PAGE 184

18 MONTHS AND UP

FAMILY FOOD GUIDE AND RECIPES

Your toddler is now 18 months old and resembles a little adult more than the infant you swaddled and rocked to sleep. Your toddler has their own thoughts and desires that they can communicate through a limited but growing vocabulary and through their actions: getting into the kitchen cabinets, climbing out of the crib, or refusing to get into the car seat. Your toddler has a personality, which can be the source of a lot of joy—and challenges!

RECIPES 157

TODDLER AT THIS STAGE

Is this the same baby I met in chapter 1? This tiny human is so independent and adventurous!

DEVELOPMENTAL SKILLS

Starting around 12 months of age, your baby started trying to mimic you, and by now, they've only gotten better at this. Your toddler mirrors your facial expression while holding your hand to walk. Your choice of language could very well be repeated back to you (uh-oh). If you enjoy a food, your child wants to enjoy it. But the converse is also true—they will copy any negative reactions as well. Do your best to ensure a happy mealtime to create positive food experiences.

NUTRITIONAL NEEDS

Your schedule of three meals and two or three snacks per day remains appropriate throughout childhood. Continue to present a variety of food to meet your child's nutritional needs. Your toddler understands their hunger and fullness, particularly if you have been following the methods described in this book. Follow your child's appetite—avoid removing food before they're ready or encouraging them to eat more when they're full. Milk intake should be limited to 16 ounces of full-fat milk per day, given with meals. Limiting the amount of milk and when it's given lets your child develop an appetite between meals, which results in better nutrition overall.

WHAT TO INTRODUCE

At 18 months of age, your child can be involved in shopping and cooking activities. Use your surroundings to communicate with your toddler—discuss where foods come from and how delicious they are. Continue to create positive food associations with family meals.

FOODS AND FLAVORS

Continue to explore food alongside your child. Consider going to a local ethnic market and selecting something new. Talk to your child about the choices. Ask your toddler which color bell pepper to select or whether they want Roma or beefsteak tomatoes. Very few foods are off-limits at this point. You still need to be careful with the choking hazards until your little one is four years old (see page 7).

TOOLS AND UTENSILS

Your toddler may not be proficient with utensils yet, but with time and many (many) opportunities to model how you eat, that will change. Your toddler likely prefers your silverware to their own. Stick with smaller dessert forks and teaspoons to continue building your child's confidence with this new skill. It's also fine if they prefer to stick with the familiar utensils they've been enjoying. They may need your assistance until three or four years of age. To help the process along, be sure to provide easily forkable foods. Anything that can be scooped, like mashed potatoes, or stabbed, like nuggets, will be great for practice.

TYPICAL MEALS AND SCHEDULE

Appropriate portion sizes for your toddler continue to be the size of their fist. A typical meal for an 18-month-old child might consist of three items—for example, a hard-boiled egg, a mini Popeye Muffin (page 157), and cucumber rounds. A typical snack might include one or two items, like a Pumpkin-Oat Breakfast Cookie (page 166) and applesauce.

Although each family will follow a different schedule, a typical schedule for this stage might look like this (see the Resources on page 189 for a link to alternative schedules).

DEALING WITH PICKY PALATES

Food neophobia is very common around this age (see Common Challenges in chapter 5 on page 118). Here are the best things you can do to guide your child toward a lifetime of food enjoyment:

AVOID CALLING YOUR CHILD "PICKY": They'll own it. And then you'll be in trouble. If you must use a term, go with something softer, like "selective."

DIVIDE THE RESPONSIBILITY: You are in charge of what is served, where it is served, and when it is served. Your child is in charge

6:00 A.M.	Wake up
6:30 A.M.	Breakfast, including 2 to 3 ounces of whole milk
9:15 A.M.	Snack, including 2 to 3 ounces of whole milk
11:30 A.M.	Lunch, including 2 to 3 ounces of whole milk
12:00 P.M.	Nap (1½ to 2 hours or more)
2:30 P.M.	Snack, including 2 to 3 ounces of whole milk
5:00 P.M.	Dinner, including 2 to 3 ounces of whole milk
6:00 P.M.	Bedtime

of whether they eat and how much they eat. See the Resources section (page 189) for further guidance.

LOOK UP, NOT DOWN: Mealtime is a time to enjoy each other. Appreciate your child's smile and growing vocabulary. Ignore their plate.

TREAT YOUR CHILD AS YOU WOULD TREAT A GUEST AT YOUR TABLE: Avoid saying anything you wouldn't say to a guest ("If you eat all your broccoli, you can have dessert").

KNOW THAT NUTRITION ISN'T A SHORT GAME: Nutritional needs are not met in one meal or even in one day. Nutritional needs are met over a few days.

The number one indicator of your child's nutritional status is the growth chart. But your gut instinct is important. If you feel that your child's accepted foods are limited, consider consulting a pediatric dietitian. Additionally, see the Resources section (page 189) for a fantastic online course that targets this concern. Let your pediatrician know if your child's selective nature is coupled with dislike of loud noises, strong smells, or noted texture aversions (such as to certain types of clothing).

Food neophobia is a normal phase that children go through. By taking a deep breath

and maintaining a positive table environment, you can ensure a healthy relationship with food moving forward.

COMMON CHALLENGES

YOUR CHILD DOESN'T LIKE MEAT: It's common for children to choose a vegetarian style of eating. Meat can seem very dry to little mouths. Try recipes that combine cooked meat with a rich sauce, like Baked Spaghetti with Meatballs (page 182), to counteract that dry feeling. Protein needs are often overstated in current media. There are plenty of nonmeat sources of protein—beans, tofu, pasta, smoothies, yogurt, nut or seed butter, cheese, milk, and eggs—that can help your child meet their nutritional needs during this phase. Continue to serve the meals you prepare for the whole family but also provide a safe dish you know your child will accept at mealtime.

YOUR CHILD LOVES TO SNACK ALL DAY LONG: Your toddler's sense of independence is growing, and it's important to honor that independence while maintaining a schedule. Why is a schedule so important? For a child to meet their nutritional needs during mealtime, they need to come to the table a little bit hungry. If your child is grazing throughout the day, they won't be hungry at mealtime. There are three easy steps to take in this scenario:

* Get a cheap clock with a white paper background. Color in wedges on the clock to represent mealtimes and other significant times, like bath time and bedtime.

* Move snacks out of your child's reach.

* Be consistent with the schedule; children thrive on predictability.

When it's snack time, present two options to your toddler. Giving your child options gives a sense of independence within healthy boundaries, which supports both their confidence and growth.

POPEYE MUFFINS

GLUTEN-FREE OPTION **NUT-FREE** VEGETARIAN VEGAN OPTION

YIELDS 12 MUFFINS

2 cups whole-wheat flour (gluten-free flour optional)

¾ cup sugar

2 teaspoons baking powder

½ teaspoon baking soda

1½ teaspoons ground cinnamon

½ teaspoon salt

¼ cup light olive oil or avocado oil, plus more for greasing

¾ cup milk (milk alternative for vegan option)

6 ounces baby spinach, tightly packed (about 3 cups)

½ cup mashed banana (about 1 large banana or 2 small bananas)

2 teaspoons vanilla extract

I'm not a fan of hiding veggies in food. Kids need to know they are eating—and enjoying—vegetables. In these muffins, there is no hiding the bright green spinach. Invite your child into the kitchen to add the ingredients to the blender and stir and scoop the batter into muffin cups. Each muffin has about ¼ cup of spinach!

1. Preheat the oven to 350°F.

2. In a large bowl, whisk together the flour, sugar, baking powder, baking soda, cinnamon, and salt. Set aside.

3. In a blender, purée the oil, milk, spinach, banana, and vanilla.

4. Pour the puréed mixture into the dry mixture and fold together with a rubber spatula until completely combined.

CONTINUED

5. Prepare a muffin tin by lightly greasing the cups with olive oil or lining the cups with paper liners. Fill each muffin cup about two-thirds full and bake 18 to 20 minutes, or until a toothpick inserted into the center comes out clean.

TO REFRIGERATE: Store in a sealed container for 3 to 5 days.

TO FREEZE: Store in an airtight container for up to 6 months.

COOKING TIP: For the sugar, you can use white sugar, brown sugar, coconut sugar, or 10 Medjool dates (soaked and blended).

CHANGE IT UP: Add some magic sprinkles on top of the muffins. You can top them with almond meal, flax meal, chopped nuts, dark chocolate chips, or shredded coconut.

SUPER BEET COOKIES

NUT-FREE VEGAN

YIELDS 8 SERVINGS

1 cup whole-wheat pastry flour or all-purpose white flour

½ teaspoon baking powder

¼ teaspoon cinnamon

¼ teaspoon salt

¾ cup shredded fresh beets (about 1 small beet)

¼ cup light olive oil, avocado oil, or coconut oil

3 large Medjool dates, pitted and mashed with a fork

¼ teaspoon vanilla extract

TO FREEZE: Store in an airtight container for up to 3 months.

Beets are an amazing source of sweet and earthy flavor, and they provide some surprising nutrition. By exposing kids of this age to unexpected flavors, you can guide them toward an appreciation that will last them a lifetime. Remember that beets stain! Consider wearing gloves and making this a diapers-only activity if kids are joining you. Parchment paper makes these much easier to roll out, and cookie cutters add to the fun. Be sure to use fresh beets, since canned beets have a different moisture content and will not work for these cookies.

1. Preheat the oven to 400°F.

2. Combine the flour, baking powder, cinnamon, and salt in a mixing bowl. Add the beets and stir. Add the oil, dates, and vanilla. Stir.

3. Knead the dough until it is smooth and the consistency of playdough.

4. Place the ball of dough on parchment paper. Cover with a second sheet of parchment and roll out to about ½ inch thick.

5. Cut out fun shapes with cookie cutters and bake the cookies on a baking sheet lined with parchment paper for 15 to 17 minutes.

6. Let cool and enjoy!

TO REFRIGERATE: Store in a sealed container for 2 to 3 days.

AVOCADO AND GRAPEFRUIT SALSA

GLUTEN-FREE **NUT-FREE** VEGAN

YIELDS 6 SERVINGS

1 grapefruit,
peeled, sectioned,
and chopped

1 avocado, peeled,
pitted, and cubed

½ cucumber, chopped

1 mini sweet
pepper, chopped

⅓ cup finely chopped
red onion

Juice of 1 lime (about
2 tablespoons)

½ teaspoon sea salt or
kosher salt

We often assume that kids want sweet flavors, but it's so important to remember that their tiny taste buds pick up the most subtle flavors. The creamy feel of avocado paired with the tang of fresh grapefruit gives this salsa a flavorful edge.

Combine the grapefruit, avocado, cucumber, sweet pepper, onion, lime juice, and salt in a bowl and mix gently. Enjoy!

TO REFRIGERATE: Store in a sealed container for up to 3 days.

CHANGE IT UP: Add ¼ teaspoon of cumin and/or ¼ cup of chopped cilantro to make this salsa something special.

SAFETY TIP: Cilantro should be well washed. I like to give it a bath in a veggie wash and then rinse thoroughly.

DIP IT!

GLUTEN-FREE **NUT-FREE** **VEGETARIAN**

Kids love to dip. Often we default to ketchup or maple syrup for dipping sauces, but there are so many more dips to try! Tzatziki (page 161), Guacamole (page 161), and Hummus (page 89) are a few of my favorites. Make a dip tray and allow your child the freedom to experience different flavors and textures. For the tzatziki, dice fresh dill by separating the soft, feathery sections of the leaves and stems from the thick stems. Roll the leaves and soft stems into a ball, then chop carefully.

TZATZIKI

YIELDS 3 SERVINGS

¾ cup plain full-fat Greek yogurt

½ cucumber, peeled, seeded, and finely chopped

2 teaspoons diced fresh dill weed, or ½ teaspoon dried dill

1½ teaspoons lemon juice

1 garlic clove, minced, or 1 teaspoon jarred minced garlic

Pinch salt

Pinch pepper

Combine the yogurt, cucumber, dill, lemon juice, garlic, salt, and pepper in a bowl and mix well.

TO REFRIGERATE: Store in an airtight container for 3 to 4 days. Freezing isn't recommended since it causes the cucumbers to lose their crunch and release liquid.

GUACAMOLE

YIELDS 3 SERVINGS

1 avocado

1 garlic clove, minced, or 1 teaspoon jarred minced garlic

¼ teaspoon lime juice (about 1 wedge)

Pinch kosher salt

CHANGE IT UP: Add a pinch of cumin, a shake of chili powder, 1 tablespoon of diced onion, and/or half a diced Roma tomato. Experiment and make this dip your own!

1. Open the avocado, remove the pit and set it aside. Scoop out the flesh with a spoon.

2. Smash the avocado with a fork, then mix in the garlic, lime juice, and salt. Enjoy!

TO REFRIGERATE: Place the avocado pit in a sealed container with the guacamole—this easy trick keeps it from browning. Keep for up to 2 days.

TO FREEZE: Pack the guacamole into a freezer-safe zip-top bag. Remove all the air and seal tightly. Freeze for 3 to 4 months.

CHICKPEA BLONDIES

GLUTEN-FREE **NUT-FREE** VEGETARIAN VEGAN OPTION

**YIELDS 12
SERVINGS**

Olive oil or butter for greasing

1 (15.5-ounce) can chickpeas, drained and rinsed

1 banana

⅓ cup sunflower seed butter

¼ cup maple syrup

¼ cup milk (milk alternative for vegan option)

1 teaspoon vanilla extract

¼ teaspoon baking powder

¼ teaspoon baking soda

¼ teaspoon salt

CHANGE IT UP:
Swap the sunflower seed butter for peanut butter or cashew butter. Replace the maple syrup with 4 or 5 soaked and pitted Medjool dates.

Chickpeas can be used to make a savory dip, like Hummus (page 89) or a sweet treat, like these blondies. Chickpeas are a great source of brain-boosting folate, tummy-supporting fiber, and multiple bone-strengthening micronutrients. Make a batch of these for a snack at home or on the go, and consider inviting your child to help add the ingredients! You'll need a food processor or a strong blender for this recipe.

1. Preheat the oven to 350°F.

2. Prepare an 8-by-8-inch baking pan by lightly coating it with olive oil or butter.

3. Place the chickpeas, banana, sunflower seed butter, maple syrup, milk, vanilla, baking powder, baking soda, and salt in the food processor. If you're using a blender, add the liquid ingredients first.

4. Blend until smooth, then pour into the prepared baking pan.

5. Bake for 25 to 30 minutes.

6. Let the blondies cool in the pan, cut into squares, and enjoy!

TO REFRIGERATE: Store in a sealed container for 3 to 4 days.

TO FREEZE: Store in an airtight container for 3 to 4 months.

PANCAKE BREAKFAST SANDWICHES

NUT-FREE **VEGETARIAN**

YIELDS 4 SERVINGS

FOR THE PANCAKES

1¼ cups all-purpose flour, sifted

1 teaspoon baking powder

¼ teaspoon sea salt

2 large eggs

1½ cups buttermilk

3 tablespoons cooking oil

1 tablespoon maple syrup

1 teaspoon vanilla extract

1 tablespoon butter

FOR THE SANDWICHES

1 tablespoon butter

4 large eggs

Pinch salt

Pinch pepper

4 slices cheese

Maple syrup, for topping

These sandwiches freeze well, so consider making extra for another day. For a heartier sandwich, top with your favorite breakfast meats, such as Canadian bacon, fully cooked sausage patties, or bacon.

TO MAKE THE PANCAKES

1. Combine the flour, baking powder, and sea salt in a medium bowl. Mix well.

2. In a separate bowl, combine the eggs, buttermilk, oil, maple syrup, and vanilla. Whisk well to mix.

3. Add the liquid ingredients to the flour mixture, taking care not to overmix. Let the batter stand for 5 minutes to rest.

4. In a skillet over medium heat, melt the butter.

5. Scoop ¼ cup of batter into the skillet to make 1 pancake. Cook until bubbles start to form on top. Flip and cook on the other side until golden brown. Continue making pancakes until you have a total of 8.

CONTINUED

TO MAKE THE SANDWICHES

1. In a separate skillet, melt the butter. Crack the eggs into the skillet, breaking the yolks with a spatula. Season with salt and pepper.

2. Flip the eggs when the whites are no longer clear and cook on the other side to desired doneness.

3. Top the eggs with cheese while they're still hot.

4. To assemble, place one pancake on a plate and drizzle with syrup. Add an egg and cheese.

5. Drizzle another pancake with maple syrup and invert onto the egg. Enjoy hot.

TO REFRIGERATE: Store separately in sealed containers for up to 5 days. Assemble just prior to serving.

TO FREEZE: Store the pancakes in an airtight container. Defrost them in the refrigerator overnight or by microwaving for 15 seconds. Cook the eggs the day you'll be serving them, then assemble the sandwiches.

SALMON AND CHEESE QUICHE

NUT-FREE

YIELDS 6 TO 8 SERVINGS

5 large eggs

1 cup milk

1 cup heavy cream

¼ teaspoon salt

Pinch pepper

1 teaspoon minced fresh dill

1 prepared pie crust

8 ounces cooked or smoked salmon

1½ cups sharp white Cheddar cheese

1 cup spinach

¼ cup sun-dried tomatoes

SAFETY TIP: Babies should not eat fish that is known to have high levels of mercury. Avoid fresh or frozen tuna, shark, swordfish, marlin, orange roughy, and canned albacore tuna.

Quiche can pack a nutritional punch, and it refrigerates and freezes nicely. When selecting a premade crust for your quiche, look for one that is "ready to bake." Carefully read the instructions on the package as some are ready to be filled and some need to be baked before filling. Have a tea party with your little one, and don't forget—pinkies up!

1. Preheat the oven to 350°F.

2. In a small bowl, whisk together the eggs, milk, and cream. Season with the salt, pepper, and dill.

3. In the pie crust, layer the salmon, cheese, spinach, and tomatoes.

4. Pour the egg filling into the crust, filling the pie crust to the top. Gently stir with a fork to mix well.

5. Bake for 45 minutes.

6. Let the quiche cool for 1½ hours before serving.

TO REFRIGERATE: Store in a sealed container for up to 5 days. Reheat at 350°F for 20 minutes in the oven or for 3 minutes in the microwave.

TO FREEZE: Store in an airtight container for up to 2 months. Defrost fully before reheating in the oven.

COOKING TIP: Substitute salmon for milder, flaked whitefish, like haddock, pollack, or flounder.

CHANGE IT UP: Experiment with different mild white cheeses. Brie, goat cheese, blue cheese, gorgonzola, feta, and Havarti are all great cheeses that melt well and change the flavor of the quiche.

PUMPKIN-OAT BREAKFAST COOKIES

GLUTEN-FREE VEGETARIAN VEGAN OPTION

YIELDS 16 COOKIES

Olive oil for greasing (optional)

2 cups old-fashioned oats

1 cup pumpkin purée

¼ cup honey or maple syrup

¼ cup flax meal

½ cup sunflower seeds

½ cup dried cranberries

2 teaspoons pumpkin spice

Pinch kosher salt

TO REFRIGERATE: Store in a sealed container for 3 to 4 days.

Jump on the breakfast-cookie train with this delicious pumpkin spice recipe, perfect for cooking with kids. Using canned pumpkin brings this recipe out of the fall and into a year-round rotation. The baking time depends on the water content of your pumpkin, so keep in mind that you may need to bake for a few minutes longer.

1. Preheat the oven to 350°F.

2. Prepare a baking sheet by lining it with a sheet of parchment paper or by lightly coating it with olive oil.

3. In a small bowl, stir the oats, pumpkin, honey, flax meal, sunflower seeds, cranberries, pumpkin spice, and salt together until they're well mixed.

4. Using a ¼-cup measuring cup, scoop the cookie dough onto the prepared baking sheet, leaving about 2 inches between cookies.

5. Bake in the oven for 10 to 12 minutes, then turn the oven off, but leave the cookies in the oven for another 10 to 12 minutes.

6. Let the cookies cool on the baking sheet and enjoy!

TO FREEZE: Store in an airtight container for 3 to 4 months.

CHANGE IT UP:

- You can replace the cranberries with raisins.
- If you don't have pumpkin pie spice, use cinnamon. Add a small pinch of nutmeg, too, if you have it.

BLUEBERRY EMPANADAS

NUT-FREE **VEGETARIAN**

YIELDS 10 TO 12 EMPANADAS

FOR THE DOUGH

1¾ cups all-purpose flour, plus extra for dusting

1 teaspoon cornstarch

Pinch salt

2 tablespoons butter, melted

2 tablespoons cold water

1 large egg yolk, beaten

FOR THE FILLING

2 cups blueberries

1 tablespoon lemon juice

2 tablespoons honey

1 egg white

What could be more delicious than a tiny berry-filled pie? Use seasonal fruits to experiment with fillings or make savory pies with leftovers. This is a pie-in-the-sky kind of recipe. The cornstarch makes the dough very forgiving and is key to making it silky and smooth. Alternatively, you can use premade pastry dough and begin at step 3.

TO MAKE THE DOUGH

1. Mix the flour, cornstarch, and salt in a medium bowl. Add the melted butter, water, and egg yolk and mix to combine. The dough should be soft.

2. In a bowl or on a clean counter, knead the dough gently until it's smooth, then wrap it in plastic wrap and chill in the refrigerator for 15 minutes.

TO MAKE THE FILLING AND ASSEMBLE EMPANANDAS

1. While the dough is chilling, place a small saucepan over medium heat. Sauté the blueberries with the lemon juice and honey until thick and bubbly. Set aside.

2. Place parchment paper on a counter and dust it with flour.

3. Transfer the chilled dough to the parchment paper and flatten into a square by rolling it up and down. Continue rolling and rotating the parchment paper 90 degrees to complete the square.

CONTINUED

4. Cut the dough into 5 or 6 palm-size squares, then cut into squares again, making 10 to 12 squares.

5. Move the parchment paper to a baking sheet and preheat the oven to 350°F.

6. Carefully spoon the blueberry filling onto one side of the dough. Moisten the other edge of the dough with a wet finger and fold it over to meet the other edge. Seal the edges with a fork or your fingers, pressing gently.

7. Create an egg wash by beating the egg white with 1 tablespoon of water. Brush the tops of the empanadas with the egg wash.

8. Bake for 12 to 15 minutes, until the tops are lightly browned.

9. Move the parchment paper to a wire rack to cool.

CHANGE IT UP:
• Try peeled and cored apples, peaches, or plums for the filling. Leftover prepared fillings taste great atop overnight oats or in yogurt or cottage cheese.
• Try the flavors of a leftover curry, beef stew, or roasted meat with vegetables.

SAFETY TIP: Fillings should be cut into bite-size portions to prevent choking.

TO REFRIGERATE: Store in a sealed container for up to 7 days. Enjoy cold or reheat in the oven or microwave until warm.

TO FREEZE: Wrap the empanadas in parchment paper and store in an airtight container for up to 3 months. Defrost in the refrigerator, then reheat in the oven at 350°F for 5 to 7 minutes or in the microwave on 50 percent power until warm.

CARROT CAKE BELGIAN WAFFLES

NUT-FREE VEGETARIAN

YIELDS 4
LARGE WAFFLES

1 cup whole-wheat flour

¾ cup rolled oats

1 tablespoon baking powder

2 teaspoons cinnamon

¼ cup cornstarch

Pinch nutmeg

¼ teaspoon salt

2 large eggs

3 tablespoons maple syrup

1½ teaspoons vanilla extract

½ cup light olive oil, coconut oil, or avocado oil

1¾ cups milk

3 medium carrots, shredded

My two-year-old twins joined me in this adventure as I crossed a recipe for comforting Belgian waffles with soft and delicious carrot cake. The result was a high-fiber and micronutrient-rich breakfast that can be eaten right away, frozen for later, or even made into a sandwich with a bit of cream cheese. You'll need to dust off your waffle maker for this one.

1. In a large bowl, mix together the flour, oats, baking powder, cinnamon, cornstarch, nutmeg, and salt.

2. Add the eggs, maple syrup, vanilla, oil, and milk to the dry ingredients.

3. Mix just to incorporate—don't overmix.

4. Fold in the carrots.

5. Using about ⅓ cup of batter for a regular waffle iron or ¾ cup of batter for a Belgian-style waffle maker, cook the batter in a waffle iron for about 3 minutes.

TO REFRIGERATE: Store in a sealed container for 3 to 4 days. Toast before enjoying.

TO FREEZE: Store in an airtight container for 3 to 4 months. Toast directly from the freezer.

COOKING TIP: If you're using a food processor to shred the carrots, allow your little one to put the carrots into the top. Little hands can also mix the batter.

CHANGE IT UP: Add one of these ingredients at step 4: a handful of raisins, dried cranberries, seeds, or chopped nuts.

PANCAKE MUFFINS

GLUTEN-FREE OPTION VEGETARIAN VEGAN OPTION

YIELDS 12 MUFFINS

Olive oil or butter for greasing (optional)

2 cups whole-wheat flour (gluten-free flour optional)

1 cup almond meal or almond flour

1 teaspoon salt

⅓ cup sugar

2½ cups milk (milk alternative for vegan option)

2 large eggs (flax eggs for vegan option)

1½ cups oil or melted butter

2 tablespoons baking powder

½ cup add-ins (see tips)

CHANGE IT UP:
Try adding ½ cup of blueberries, strawberries, raspberries, chopped peaches, or bananas, or ½ cup total of cheese and sausage bits.

This is my favorite pancake recipe, but you can certainly use your own favorite batter recipe or pancake mix to make quick and delicious pancake muffins. Whether you choose homemade or semi-homemade, the key is the add-ins. Pancake muffins are wonderful for breakfast or for a snack at home or on the go. Involve the kids by setting out add-in options and allowing them to make their own pancake muffin creations.

1. Preheat the oven to 425°F.

2. Prepare a muffin tin by lining the cups with paper or silicone liners or lightly coating them with olive oil or butter.

3. Whisk together the flour, almond meal, salt, sugar, milk, eggs, and oil until well mixed.

4. Sprinkle in the baking powder and add-ins and mix to incorporate.

5. If the batter is too thick, add more milk, 1 tablespoon at a time, to achieve the desired consistency.

6. Fill the muffin cups three-quarters full.

7. Bake for 20 minutes, or until golden. Remove the muffins from the oven, let cool, then enjoy!

TO REFRIGERATE: Store in a sealed container for up to 4 days.

TO FREEZE: Store in an airtight container for up to 4 months.

BURST TOMATOES AND PASTA

GLUTEN-FREE OPTION **NUT-FREE** VEGAN

YIELDS 4 SERVINGS

2 tablespoons olive oil, plus extra for greasing

2 (10-ounce) containers cherry tomatoes

6 garlic cloves, minced, or 6 teaspoons jarred minced garlic

1 teaspoon kosher salt

4 ounces whole-grain pasta, prepared according to package instructions (gluten-free pasta optional)

TO REFRIGERATE: Store in a sealed container for 3 to 4 days.

From spaghetti, rotini, and ziti, to vegetable noodles made with a spiralizer, kids love pasta. A great way to incorporate a fun veggie is to add burst cherry tomatoes. When a vegetable is cooked, natural sugars are released, resulting in a sweeter flavor that's often more palatable to kids (and many adults). Serve these garlic-roasted cherry tomatoes on pasta or as a side dish with toast points and creamy goat cheese.

1. Preheat the oven to 375°F.

2. Prepare a baking sheet by lining it with foil and lightly coating it with olive oil.

3. In a small bowl, mix the tomatoes with the garlic, 2 tablespoons of olive oil, and salt.

4. Lay the tomatoes on the baking sheet in a single, even layer.

5. Bake for 20 to 25 minutes.

6. Toss the tomatoes in the pasta, let cool, and enjoy!

SAFETY TIP: Cherry and grape tomatoes usually should be halved prior to serving them to small children, but these are roasted, so the cooking eliminates the safety risk. You can halve your tomatoes for this recipe if you wish.

CHICKEN PESTO PASTA

GLUTEN-FREE OPTION **NUT-FREE**

YIELDS 4 TO 6 SERVINGS

2 cups spinach, leaves only

¼ cup fresh basil

3 garlic cloves, minced, divided

¼ cup olive oil, plus 1 tablespoon

¼ cup shredded Parmesan cheese, plus more for garnish

1 shallot, minced

2 pounds boneless, skinless chicken breasts or thighs, cubed

8 ounces pasta, cooked according to package instructions (gluten-free pasta optional)

Salt

Spinach has a mild flavor that is complemented by garlic and basil. It is naturally high in folate, an essential B vitamin. This recipe tastes even better the next day, after the flavors have had the chance to mature.

1. Place the spinach, basil, and 1 garlic clove in a food processor and purée until smooth.

2. Slowly add ¼ cup of olive oil, 1 tablespoon at a time, pulsing the mixture after each addition.

3. Add the Parmesan cheese and pulse to mix. Place the pesto in a large bowl and set aside.

4. Heat the remaining 1 tablespoon of olive oil in a shallow pan over medium heat. Sauté the remaining 2 garlic cloves and the shallot for 2 minutes, until fragrant. Add the chicken and cook until browned, 5 to 7 minutes.

5. Toss warm, cooked pasta and chicken with the pesto to mix.

6. Season with salt and top with grated Parmesan to serve.

TO REFRIGERATE: Store in a sealed container for up to 3 days.

TO FREEZE: Store in an airtight container for up to 2 months. Defrost in the refrigerator overnight and reheat in the microwave on 50 percent power to warm.

COOKING TIP: When draining your pasta, save a few tablespoons of the cooking water. If your pesto is too thick, this water is ideal for using to thin the sauce.

CHANGE IT UP: The pesto can be made more traditionally using only basil, but the spinach helps reduce the cost of homemade pesto while retaining its flavor.

YELLOW CURRY WITH CHICKEN

GLUTEN-FREE **NUT-FREE**

YIELDS 6 (1-CUP) SERVINGS

Curry can often have strong flavors, so double-check yours to make sure it has the heat level you want. Adding coconut milk mellows the flavor and adds a creamy and comforting texture. To thicken, mash a few of the white potatoes against the inside of the pot and mix. This dish tastes even better the next day, once the flavors have intensified.

1 tablespoon yellow curry powder

1 teaspoon sea salt

1 tablespoon avocado oil or other cooking oil

½ cup diced onion

2 garlic cloves, minced

1 teaspoon minced ginger

1½ pounds boneless, skiness chicken breasts or thighs, cubed

½ cup diced white potatoes

½ cup diced carrots

1 cup low-sodium chicken broth

1¼ cups canned coconut milk

½ cup broccoli florets

1 Roma tomato, diced

Rice or riced cauliflower, steamed, for serving

Chopped cilantro, for garnish (optional)

Chopped cashews, for garnish (optional)

TO FREEZE: Store in an airtight container for up to 6 months. Thaw in the refrigerator overnight. Reheat on medium heat until heated throughout.

TO REFRIGERATE: Store in a sealed container for up to 3 days.

1. Put the curry powder and salt in a 4-quart pot over medium heat. Heat for 1 minute, stirring continuously.

2. Add the oil, onion, garlic, and ginger. Sauté for 1 minute, until fragrant.

3. Add the chicken and cook until browned, about 5 minutes.

4. Add the potatoes and carrots. Sauté for 1 minute.

5. Add the chicken broth, cover, and cook for 10 minutes.

6. Add the coconut milk, mixing well.

7. Add the broccoli and tomato. Cover and cook for 3 to 4 minutes or to desired texture.

8. Serve hot over rice or riced cauliflower. Garnish with chopped cilantro and cashews, if using.

BABY-LED FEEDING TIP: When dicing vegetables, aim for a toddler bite–size piece. Children are more likely to try something that looks like a small bite rather than something they have to bite into pieces.

SAFETY TIP: Wash the cilantro thoroughly before use.

CHANGE IT UP: I use chicken thighs for this dish. The dark meat is higher in iron and more flavorful overall.

COOKING TIP: Riced cauliflower is readily available in both fresh and frozen packages with clear instructions at most grocery stores.

LASAGNA ROLL-UP

NUT FREE VEGETARIAN

YIELDS 8 TO
10 ROLLS

4 lasagna noodles

1 cup ricotta cheese

¾ cup grated
Parmesan cheese

1 large egg, beaten

¼ teaspoon salt

¼ teaspoon
black pepper

1 (15-ounce) jar
Alfredo sauce

1 cup pesto from
Chicken Pesto Pasta
(page 172)

Rolled lasagna changes the presentation of a classic lasagna. The Alfredo sauce and pesto flavors are elevated with the cheeses. This recipe is tomato-free for those trying to consume less acid. This recipe can also be made using the Veggieful Sauce (page 73).

1. Preheat the oven to 350°F.

2. Gently boil the lasagna noodles in salted water for 5 to 7 minutes, until just pliable. Do not overcook. Allow the noodles to dry on warmed dish towels.

3. Combine the ricotta, Parmesan, egg, salt, and black pepper in a small bowl and mix with a fork to combine. Set aside.

4. Layer ¼ cup of Alfredo sauce in a 9-by-12-inch baking dish. Set aside.

5. Using scissors, cut each noodle in half (widthwise) to yield 8 equally sized noodles.

6. Spread the ricotta mixture across each noodle. Add a layer of pesto on top.

7. Roll up each noodle gently. Filling may spill out the sides if the noodle is wrapped too tightly. Gently press any extra filling back into the noodles if necessary.

8. Place the roll-ups in the baking dish, seam-side down, and top with the remaining Alfredo sauce. Bake for 30 to 35 minutes.

9. Remove from the oven and serve hot.

TO REFRIGERATE: Store in a sealed container for up to 5 days.

TO FREEZE: Stop after step 7 and store in an airtight container (with or without sauce) for up to 2 months. Allow to fully defrost before baking at 350°F for 40 to 45 minutes.

COOKING TIP: A store-bought pesto can be substituted for the homemade sauce.

CHANGE IT UP: Add some diced leftover chicken and sun-dried tomatoes or a layer of spinach or another soft, leafy green.

MOROCCAN LENTIL AND CHICKPEA SOUP

GLUTEN-FREE **NUT-FREE** VEGAN

**YIELDS 4 TO 5
(1-CUP) SERVINGS**

1 tablespoon olive oil,
plus more for drizzling

1 onion, diced

2 teaspoons berbere
seasoning

1 (15-ounce) can
diced tomatoes

1 teaspoon sugar

½ cup yellow lentils

3⅔ cups low-sodium
vegetable broth

½ cup chickpeas,
drained

½ cup frozen baby
lima beans

1 teaspoon salt

1 teaspoon
black pepper

½ tablespoon
chopped fresh
cilantro, for garnish

½ tablespoon
chopped fresh
parsley, for garnish

Berbere is an Ethiopian spice blend that adds warmth and depth of flavor to the lentils in this soup. Cooking the spice for just a minute before adding the tomatoes releases some of the spice's aromatic oils, intensifying the flavor. This dish is even better reheated the next day, when the flavors have fully set.

1. Heat the oil in a 4-quart pot over medium heat. Add the onion and sauté for 2 minutes.

2. Add the berbere, the tomatoes, including the juice, and the sugar.

3. Add the lentils and broth. Bring to a boil, then reduce heat to low. Simmer for 20 minutes.

4. Stir in the chickpeas and lima beans. Simmer for 5 minutes more.

5. Add the salt and pepper. Serve garnished with a drizzle of olive oil, cilantro, and parsley.

TO REFRIGERATE: Store in a sealed container for up to 1 week. Reheat in the microwave or over medium heat on the stove.

TO FREEZE: Store in an airtight container for up to 2 months. Defrost in the refrigerator overnight. Reheat in the microwave or over medium heat on the stove.

COOKING TIP: Berbere is a flavorful blend of spices used in traditional Ethiopian cuisine. If you can't find it in your local grocery store, combine ½ teaspoon of paprika, ¼ teaspoon of cinnamon, ½ teaspoon of garlic powder, and ¼ teaspoon of ginger.

LOADED BAKED SWEET POTATO BAR

GLUTEN-FREE **NUT-FREE** VEGETARIAN VEGAN OPTION

YIELDS 4 SERVINGS

4 sweet potatoes

2 tablespoons olive oil

3 tablespoons butter (butter alternative for vegan option)

2 garlic cloves, minced

¼ teaspoon salt

¾ cup shredded cheese, for topping (cheese alternative for vegan option)

2 tablespoons minced chives, for topping

CHANGE IT UP:
You had me at sweet! Replace the garlic, salt, and shredded cheese with classic flavors of brown sugar, cinnamon, chopped walnuts, or cranberries.

Nothing releases all the natural sweetness of a sweet potato like baking. Combining your favorite toppings in a self-serve style gets the whole family involved, and mixing savory toppings with the sweet potato provides the ultimate umami flavor. Consider avocado chunks, bacon crumbles, cheese, chives, or garlic butter with parsley.

1. Preheat the oven to 350°F.

2. Wash the sweet potatoes and pat dry. Poke each potato all over with a fork.

3. Rub each potato with the oil and wrap in aluminum foil.

4. Bake the potatoes on a baking sheet for 20 minutes until tender and soft to the touch. Set aside and let cool.

5. Melt the butter in a shallow pan over medium heat. Add the garlic and sauté for 2 minutes. Add the salt and turn off the heat.

6. Unwrap the cooled potatoes. Slice each one down the center.

7. Gently squeeze the potato at the middle on each side to release the potato from its skin.

8. Drizzle the potatoes with the garlic butter. Place the cheese, chives, and other toppings in small bowls and serve with the potatoes.

TO REFRIGERATE: Store for up to 5 days in an airtight container. Gently reheat in the microwave before topping.

BREADSTICKS

GLUTEN-FREE OPTION | **NUT-FREE** | VEGETARIAN

**YIELDS 12
BREADSTICKS**

FOR THE STARTER

1 package
(2¼ teaspoons)
active dry yeast

½ cup warm water

1 tablespoon honey

1 cup bread flour
(gluten-free flour
optional)

½ cup warm milk

FOR THE DOUGH

2¼ cups bread flour
(gluten-free flour
optional), plus extra
for dusting

1 teaspoon salt

1 tablespoon sugar

¼ cup grated
Parmesan cheese

4 tablespoons olive oil

1 large egg, beaten,
room temperature

Warm and satisfying, breadsticks are a great snack, and they pair perfectly with many of the recipes in this book. Dip them in the Minestrone Soup (page 140) or the Chicken Pesto Pasta (page 172).

TO MAKE THE STARTER

1. Combine the yeast, warm water, and honey in a glass bowl. Whisk well.

2. Let stand for 5 minutes.

3. Add the bread flour and milk. Stir to mix.

4. Cover the starter with a warm, dry towel and let it sit for 1 hour. It will be sticky and shapeless.

TO MAKE THE DOUGH

1. Whisk together the bread flour, salt, sugar, and Parmesan in a large mixing bowl.

2. Make a well in the center of the dry ingredients and add the starter and olive oil.

3. Using a silicone spatula, fold in the flour mixture, taking care not to overmix.

4. Turn out the dough onto a floured counter and knead it gently until it is silky and smooth.

5. Place the dough in a well-oiled bowl and cover with plastic wrap. Cover the bowl with a warm towel and let the dough rise in a draft-free space for 45 to 50 minutes.

6. Remove the dough from the bowl. It will be soft, full of air bubbles, and almost doubled in size. Punch it down and knead it a few times until it's smooth and springy.

7. Section the dough into 12 equal parts and shape it into breadstick shapes. Line a baking sheet with parchment paper. Place the breadsticks on the baking sheet. Brush the tops of the breadsticks with the beaten egg.

8. Cover the breadsticks with plastic wrap and let them rise in a draft-free space for 30 minutes. The dough will be smooth and bounce back when touched.

9. Preheat the oven to 350°F.

10. Bake the breadsticks for 30 to 35 minutes, or until golden to light brown.

TO STORE: Refrigerating bread dries out the trapped water and makes the bread stale faster. Store on the counter in an airtight container. Reheat to enjoy.

TO FREEZE: Store in an airtight container before the second rise. Defrost on a parchment paper–lined baking sheet overnight. Bake at 350°F for 40 to 45 minutes.

COOKING TIP: Garnish the top of your breadsticks with herbs, garlic powder, or dried basil before the second rise. You can even whisk some of the leftover pesto from the Chicken Pesto Pasta (page 172) together with your egg wash.

BAKED SPAGHETTI WITH MEATBALLS

GLUTEN-FREE OPTION   **NUT-FREE**

YIELDS 6 SERVINGS

FOR THE MEATBALLS

½ pound
Italian sausage

1 pound ground chuck
or ground sirloin

2 garlic cloves, minced

1 onion,
finely chopped

2 tablespoons minced
fresh parsley

1 tablespoon
dried oregano

Pinch salt

Pinch pepper

¼ cup bread crumbs
(gluten-free bread
crumbs optional)

½ cup grated
Parmesan cheese

1 large egg, beaten

Olive oil, for greasing

I love the rich creaminess of Alfredo sauce paired with marinara sauce. The sauces create an irresistible flavor. Soak it up with some Breadsticks (page 180). Both the meatballs and baked spaghetti freeze well, so make a batch for an easy meal later.

TO MAKE THE MEATBALLS

1. Preheat the oven to 350°F.

2. Combine the Italian sausage and ground chuck in a medium bowl and mix well. Add the garlic, onion, parsley, oregano, salt, and pepper. Mix well. Add the bread crumbs, Parmesan cheese, and egg. Combine until well incorporated, taking care not to overmix.

3. Portion the meat mixture into 10 to 12 balls that are each 1 to 2 inches in diameter. These will shrink during cooking. Bake for 25 to 30 minutes on a well-oiled baking sheet.

TO MAKE THE BAKED SPAGHETTI

1. Cook the pasta according to the package instructions to just under done (al dente pasta will become too soft after baking).

2. In a medium bowl, combine the Alfredo sauce, parsley, garlic, and Romano cheese. Add the pasta, tossing with a fork to mix. Let the mixture sit for 5 minutes.

3. In a well-oiled, deep baking dish, layer the spaghetti and any remaining sauce from the bowl. Bake for 25 minutes, or until the sauce is bubbly. Let the spaghetti mixture stand for 10 minutes to set.

4. While the spaghetti mixture is resting, heat the marinara sauce in a saucepan over medium heat.

5. Using a sharp knife or spatula, cut the baked spaghetti into rectangles.

6. Serve topped with marinara sauce and meatballs.

TO REFRIGERATE: Store in a sealed container for up to 5 days. Reheat on medium heat in the microwave to prevent the sauce from separating.

TO FREEZE: Store the spaghetti unbaked in an airtight container for up to 2 months. Defrost completely overnight in the refrigerator, then bake at 350°F for 40 to 45 minutes. The meatballs can be cooked and frozen for up to 2 months. Reheat the frozen meatballs in the marinara sauce as it is warming.

COOKING TIP: In a crunch for time? This dish is delicious without the meatballs and features protein from the cheeses.

FOR THE BAKED SPAGHETTI

8 ounces spaghetti (gluten-free pasta optional)

1½ cups Alfredo sauce

1 tablespoon dried parsley

1 garlic clove, minced

8 ounces Romano or Parmesan cheese, grated

Olive oil, for greasing

2 cups marinara sauce

CORNBREAD AND CHILI WAFFLE

GLUTEN-FREE OPTION **NUT-FREE**

YIELDS 6 SERVINGS

Chili is a hearty meal that's great all year. The beans are soft and easy for little ones to chew. Serve atop Cornbread (page 130) cooked on your waffle iron. Consider adding sour cream, chopped scallions, or shredded cheese and allow the cheese to melt before serving.

1 tablespoon cooking oil

½ cup chopped onion

2 garlic cloves, minced

2 teaspoons salt

2 teaspoons ground pepper

1 teaspoon paprika

½ teaspoon cumin

½ teaspoon chipotle chili powder

¼ teaspoon cayenne pepper

1 pound ground beef

½ cup carrots, diced

½ cup green bell pepper, diced

½ cup red bell pepper, diced

1 jalapeño, seeded and diced

½ cup low-sodium beef broth

½ cup canned white beans, drained and rinsed

½ cup pinto beans, drained and rinsed

½ cup red beans, drained and rinsed

1 recipe Cornbread (page 130)

TO FREEZE: Store in an airtight container for up to 2 months. Defrost overnight in the refrigerator. Reheat the chili on the stovetop until hot. Reheat the cornbread in the toaster or oven until hot.

1. Heat the cooking oil in a skillet over medium heat. Sauté the onion and garlic for 2 minutes. Add the salt, pepper, paprika, cumin, chili powder, and cayenne pepper.

2. Add the ground beef and cook until browned. Do not drain.

3. Add the carrots, green bell pepper, red bell pepper, and jalapeño. Sauté for 2 minutes. Add the broth and the white, pinto, and red beans. Simmer for 12 minutes.

4. Serve hot atop cornbread.

TO REFRIGERATE: Store the chili in a sealed container for up to 5 days. Reheat in the microwave or on the stovetop until hot. Store the cornbread at room temperature and reheat in the toaster or oven until hot.

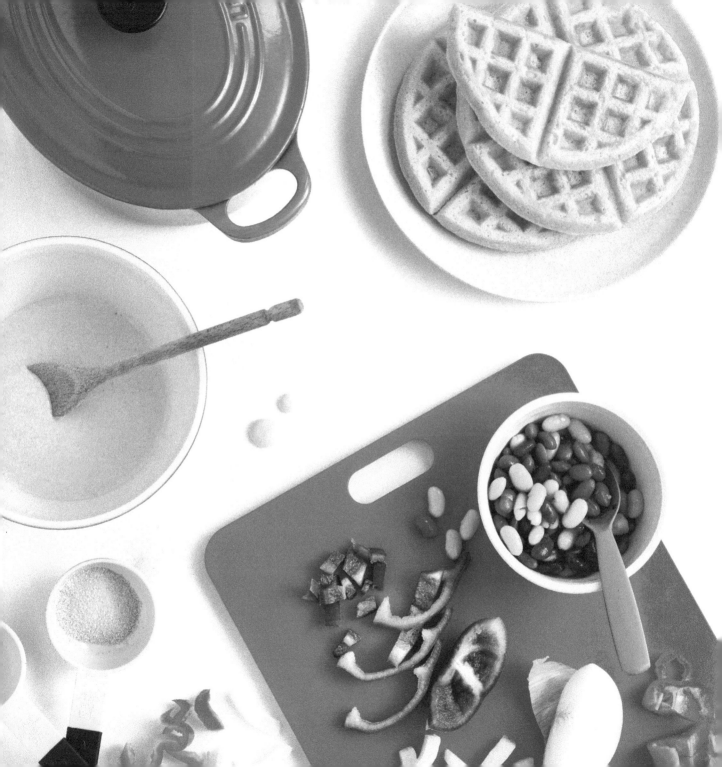

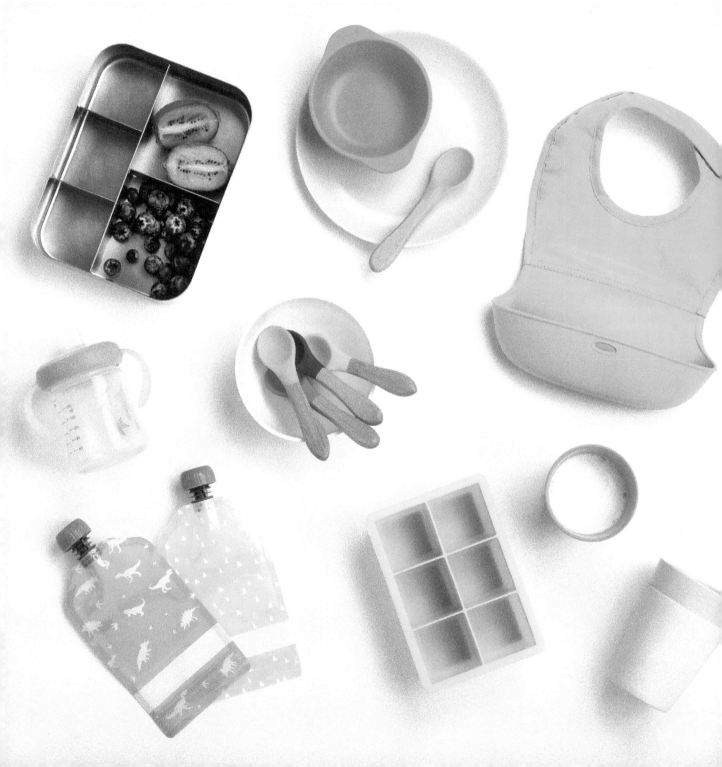

MEASUREMENT CONVERSIONS

VOLUME EQUIVALENTS (LIQUID)

US STANDARD	US STANDARD (OUNCES)	METRIC (APPROXIMATE)
2 tablespoons	1 fl. oz.	30 mL
¼ cup	2 fl. oz.	60 mL
½ cup	4 fl. oz.	120 mL
1 cup	8 fl. oz.	240 mL
1½ cups	12 fl. oz.	355 mL
2 cups or 1 pint	16 fl. oz.	475 mL
4 cups or 1 quart	32 fl. oz.	1 L
1 gallon	128 fl. oz.	4 L

OVEN TEMPERATURES

FAHRENHEIT (F)	CELSIUS (C) (APPROXIMATE)
250°F	120°C
300°F	150°C
325°F	165°C
350°F	180°C
375°F	190°C
400°F	200°C
425°F	220°C
450°F	230°C

VOLUME EQUIVALENTS (DRY)

US STANDARD	METRIC (APPROXIMATE)	US STANDARD	METRIC (APPROXIMATE)
⅛ teaspoon	0.5 mL	½ cup	118 mL
¼ teaspoon	1 mL	⅔ cup	156 mL
½ teaspoon	2 mL	¾ cup	177 mL
¾ teaspoon	4 mL	1 cup	235 mL
1 teaspoon	5 mL	2 cups or 1 pint	475 mL
1 tablespoon	15 mL	3 cups	700 mL
¼ cup	59 mL	4 cups or 1 quart	1 L
⅓ cup	79 mL		

WEIGHT EQUIVALENTS

US STANDARD	METRIC (APPROXIMATE)
½ ounce	15 g
1 ounce	30 g
2 ounces	60 g
4 ounces	115 g
8 ounces	225 g
12 ounces	340 g
16 ounces or 1 pound	455 g

REFERENCES

AMERICAN ACADEMY OF PEDIATRICS. "Starting Solid Foods." Last modified January 16, 2018. https://www.healthychildren.org/English/ages-stages/baby/feeding-nutrition/Pages/Starting-Solid-Foods.aspx.

——. "Weaning from the Bottle." Accessed October 14, 2019. https://www.aap.org/en-us/about-the-aap/aap-press-room/aap-press-room-media-center/Pages/Weaning-from-the-Bottle.aspx.

AMERICAN ACADEMY OF PEDIATRICS SECTION ON BREASTFEEDING. "Breastfeeding and the Use of Human Milk." *Pediatrics* 129, no. 3 (March 2012): e827–e841. https://doi.org/10.1542/peds.2011-3552.

BENTLEY, AMY. "Booming Baby Food: Infant Food and Feeding in Post–World War II America." *Michigan Historical Review* 32, no. 2 (Fall 2006): 63–87. https://research.steinhardt.nyu.edu/scmsAdmin/uploads/005/529/MHR%20article.pdf.

CENTERS FOR DISEASE CONTROL AND PREVENTION. "When, What, and How to Introduce Solid Foods." Last modified October 17, 2019. https://www.cdc.gov/nutrition/infantandtoddlernutrition/foods-and-drinks/when-to-introduce-solid-foods.html

——. "WHO Growth Charts." Last modified September 9, 2010. https://www.cdc.gov/growthcharts/who_charts.htm.

FOLSOM, LISAL J., AND LINDA A. DIMEGLIO. "Recommendations Released on Prevention, Management of Rickets." AAP News and Journals Gateway. February 10, 2017. https://www.aappublications.org/news/2017/02/10/Rickets021017.

GREER, FRANK R., SCOTT H. SICHERER, AND A. WESLEY BURKS. Committee on Nutrition, Section on Allergy and Immunology. *"The Effects of Early Nutritional Interventions on the Development of Atopic Disease in Infants and Children: The Role of Maternal Dietary Restriction, Breastfeeding, Hydrolyzed Formulas, and Timing of Introduction of Allergenic Complementary Foods."* Pediatrics 143, no. 4 (April 2019): e20190281. https://doi.org/10.1542/peds.2019-0281.

SÄÄTELÄ, ELSA. "BABY FOOD AROUND THE WORLD." *The Daily Meal.* November 14, 2013. https://www.thedailymeal.com/travel/baby-food-around-world-slideshow.

US FOOD AND DRUG ADMINISTRATION. "WHAT YOU NEED TO KNOW ABOUT FOOD ALLERGIES." Accessed October 11, 2019. https://www.fda.gov/food/buy-store-serve-safe-food/what-you-need-know-about-food-allergies.

WORLD HEALTH ORGANIZATION. "BREASTFEEDING." Accessed October 15, 2019. https://www.who.int/nutrition/topics/exclusive_breastfeeding/en/.

RESOURCES

NUTRITION FOR RAISING CHILDREN

NAPTIMENUTRITION.COM: You can find me weekly on my Facebook page, giving free and relevant information on parenting, children, and nutrition. Use the search tab to explore topics I've covered since 2016, including gluten, fat, pumping, how to read growth charts, and so much more!

BABY-LED FEEDING

FEEDINGLITTLES.COM: Feeding Littles has wonderful online courses on both baby-led weaning and toddler feeding.

CHILD NUTRITION

ELLYNSATTERINSTITUTE.ORG: Ellyn Satter, MS, RD, MSSW, developed the model for the division of responsibility in feeding. Her site is a valuable resource for further information on guiding your child toward a healthy relationship with food and body.

FEEDINGBYTES.COM: Natalia Stasenko, RD, is a feeding expert who provides up-to-date and convenient resources on her website and social media outlets.

THEFEEDINGDOCTOR.COM: Katja Rowell, MD, provides books, blogs, and other free resources on child nutrition, extremely picky eating, food preoccupation, and much more.

HEALTHYCHILDREN.ORG: The American Academy of Pediatrics' parenting website provides reliable health information about children and parenting.

"PREVENTION OF RICKETS AND VITAMIN D DEFICIENCY IN INFANTS, CHILDREN, AND ADOLESCENTS" by Carol L. Wagner, Frank R. Greer, and the Section on Breastfeeding and Committee on Nutrition. See the full paper at https://pediatrics.aappublications.org/content/pediatrics/122/5/1142.full.pdf to learn more about the recent recommendation for increased vitamin D supplementation in infants and children.

BABYWEARING

BABYWEARINGINTERNATIONAL.ORG: Babywearing International is an amazing resource for all things babywearing. They have trained coaches as well as a lending library. Find the chapter in your area and regain access to both hands!

TANDEMTROUBLE.COM: LaKeta Kemp, babywearing coach and twin mom (like me!), demonstrates how to safely and comfortably wear twins.

BREASTFEEDING

ILCA.ORG: The website for the International Lactation Consultant Association has a search function to help connect you with an international board-certified lactation consultant. Having an advocate during this amazing time can provide important relief.

CRYSTALKARGES.COM AND MAMAANDSWEETPEANUTRITION.COM: Find reliable and compassionate advice on breastfeeding and breastfeeding nutrition from these two registered dietitians.

SLEEPING AND FEEDING SCHEDULES

GETQUIETNIGHTS.COM: Tracy Spackman provides gentle sleep-coaching information. See her blog for daily schedules with alternative options.

INDEX

ACKNOWLEDGMENTS

This book would not have been possible without support from my family. Shimmy, Ben, and Daniel, you've been there with lots of hugs and kisses. My parents and brother, Joan, Lenny, and Brian Kalmenson, have provided constructive comments through the years. I even listened sometimes. My grandmother Phyllis Chaiken has always told me that I'm doing the right thing.

This book never would have happened without my friend and partner in trouble LaKeta Kemp. Bracha Kopstick, this would be a raw gem without your careful and insightful polishing. And of course, my fabulous editor, Laura Apperson, who made this as easy as possible.

And no mom/small businesswoman is complete without her tribe. Jessica Abbott has always been there to remind me to breathe. Shternie, Rena, Chava, Sara, Bonnie, Dina, Elisheva, Gila, Tamar, Zahava, and the rest of the group. I don't have enough words to thank you all.

Lev, you have given me love, encouragement, and the space to create. You've held my hand through this journey through school and into parenthood. I wouldn't want to do this with anyone else. You are the Lev of my life.

ABOUT THE AUTHOR

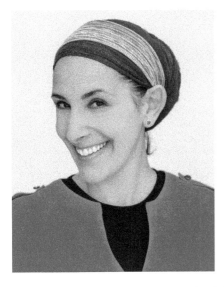

YAFFI LVOVA is a registered dietitian nutritionist and the owner of Baby Bloom Nutrition. She holds degrees in both Comparative Religions and Nutrition and Dietetics from Arizona State University.

After a difficult journey toward and into motherhood, Yaffi became mother to twins plus one. She used her experience and clinical knowledge to shift gears and help smooth the transition into parenthood for new and expecting parents by providing them with nutrition education.

In 2015, Yaffi created Toddler Test Kitchen (toddlertestkitchen.net) with immense help from Claudine Wessel, LaKeta Kemp, and Sarah Garone. This unique culinary adventure puts small children in the driver's seat—or at the cutting board as it were—which helps bolster their self-esteem as they feed their curiosity by creating something delicious!

In 2016, Yaffi went live with a weekly Facebook segment and subsequent podcast, *Nap Time Nutrition* (naptimenutrition.com), which covers all topics parenthood and nutrition.

In 2019, Yaffi was brought on board for the update of *Discover Mindful Eating for Kids* and *Stage-by-Stage Baby Food Cookbook*.

You can find Yaffi at babybloomnutrition.com. Yaffi is also on Facebook at Baby Bloom Nutrition and Toddler Test Kitchen, and on Instagram at @toddler.testkitchen.

CPSIA information can be obtained
at www.ICGtesting.com
Printed in the USA
JSHW071152140223
37549JS00003B/3

9 781641 529716